Surgical Infections - Some Facts

Edited by Manal Mohammad Baddour

Published in London, United Kingdom

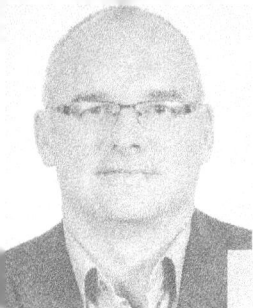
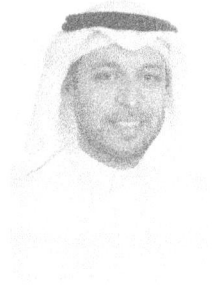
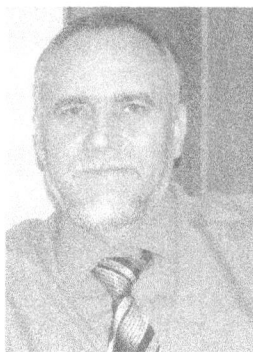
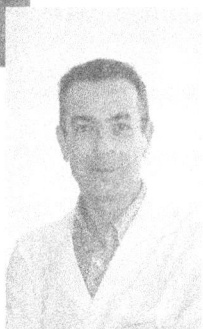
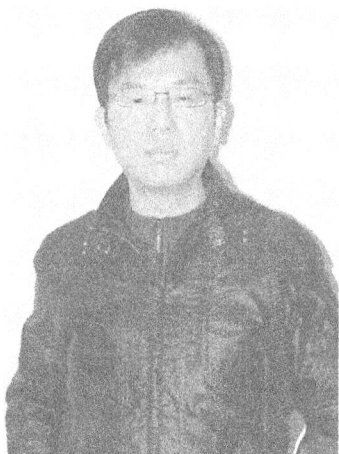
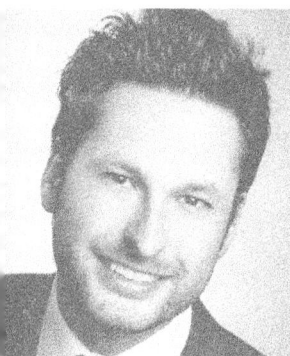
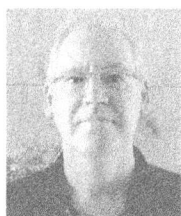

IntechOpen

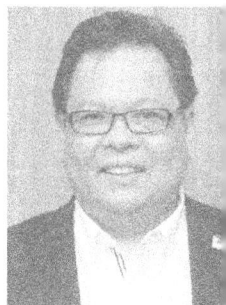
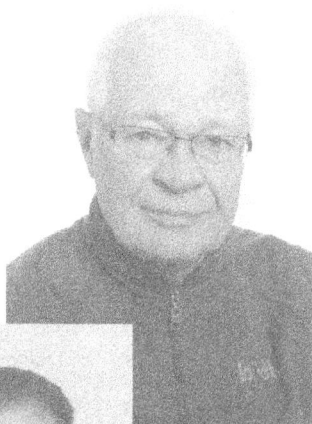
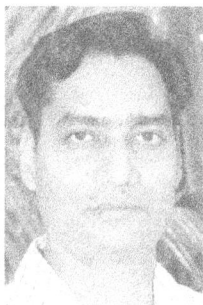
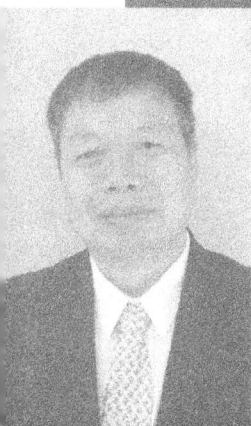
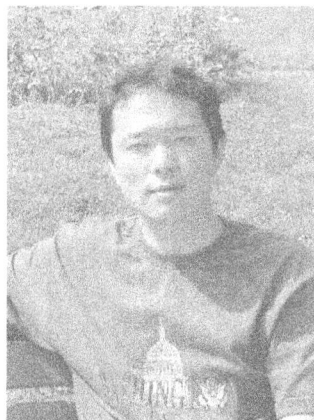
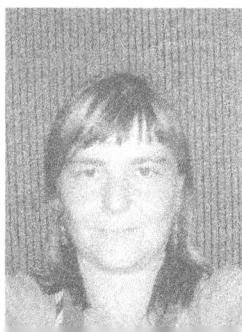

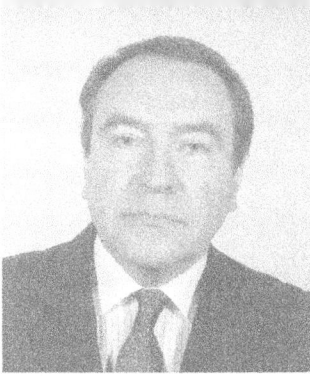

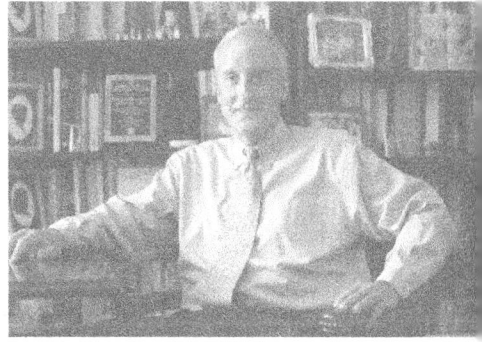

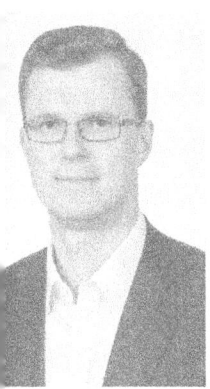

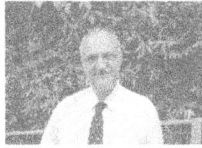

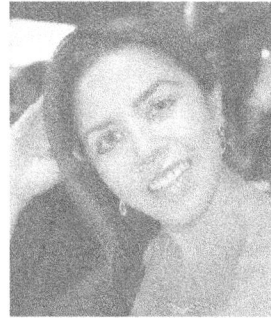

Supporting open minds since 2005

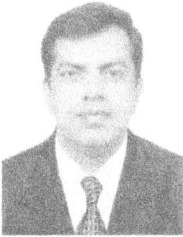

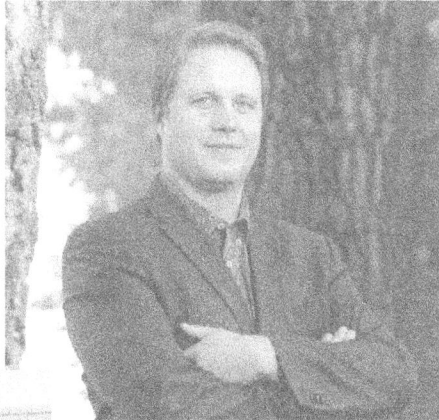

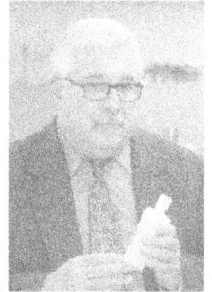

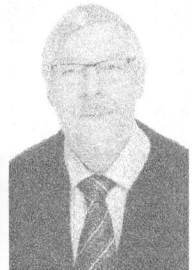

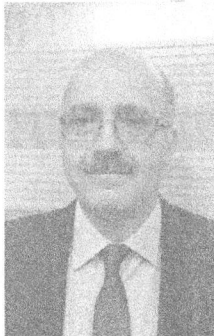

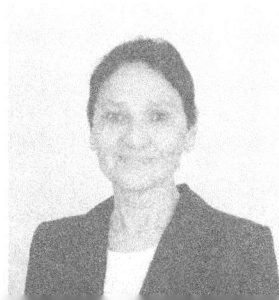

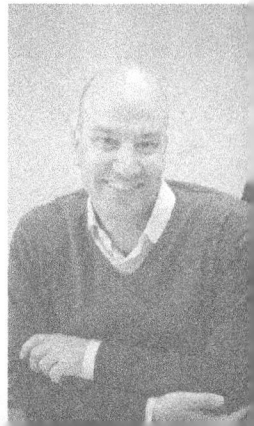

Surgical Infections - Some Facts
http://dx.doi.org/10.5772/intechopen.73852
Edited by Manal Mohammad Baddour

Contributors
Esmail Khodadadi, Livia Barenghi, Alberto Barenghi, Alberto Di Balsio, Hadir Okasha, Manal Mohammad
Baddour

Notice
Statements and opinions expressed in the chapters are these of the individual contributors and not
necessarily those of the editors or publisher. No responsibility is accepted for the accuracy of
information contained in the published chapters. The publisher assumes no responsibility for any
damage or injury to persons or property arising out of the use of any materials, instructions, methods
or ideas contained in the book.

First published in London, United Kingdom, 2020 by IntechOpen
IntechOpen is the global imprint of INTECHOPEN LIMITED, registered in England and Wales,
registration number: 11086078, 7th floor, 10 Lower Thames Street, London,
EC3R 6AF, United Kingdom
Printed in Croatia

British Library Cataloguing-in-Publication Data
A catalogue record for this book is available from the British Library

Additional hard and PDF copies can be obtained from orders@intechopen.com

Surgical Infections - Some Facts
Edited by Manal Mohammad Baddour
p. cm.
Print ISBN 978-1-83968-534-7
Online ISBN 978-1-83968-535-4
eBook (PDF) ISBN 978-1-83968-536-1

We are IntechOpen,
the world's leading publisher of
Open Access books

Built by scientists, for scientists

4,600+
Open access books available

119,000+
International authors and editors

135M+
Downloads

Our authors are among the

151
Countries delivered to

Top 1%
most cited scientists

12.2%
Contributors from top 500 universities

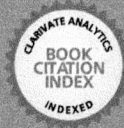

Interested in publishing with us?
Contact book.department@intechopen.com

Numbers displayed above are based on latest data collected.
For more information visit www.intechopen.com

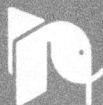

Meet the editor

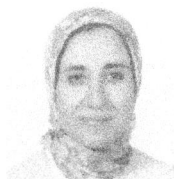

Manal Mohammad Baddour is a professor of medical microbiology and immunology in the Faculty of Medicine, Alexandria University, Egypt. She received her PhD in Microbiology and Immunology in 1995 from Alexandria University, Egypt. She ranked first on High School Examinees all over the kingdom of Saudi Arabia in 1979. She has been listed in the *Marquis Who's Who in the World* for 2009 and in the Academic Keys Who's Who list for Medicine Higher Education. She has held several positions, including Secretary General of the Permanent Scientific Committee for Promotion of Professors and Associate Professors in Medical Microbiology and Immunology, Egypt (2 rounds). She has been appointed editor/associate editor for five scientific journals, a reviewer for 19 scientific journals, as well as an assessor for promotion files of faculty members from Egyptian, Jordanian, and Saudi Arabian Universities. She has also been the editor of two books, the author of one book, and author/coauthor of 33 publications in scientific journals. She has held memberships in several organizations, including the Gerson Lehrman Group for Healthcare & Biomedical Council, Society for General Microbiology, England, Egyptian Society for Medical Microbiology, Egyptian Association of Immunologists, Egyptian Society for Infection Control, Egyptian Medical Syndicate, Alexandria Medical Syndicate, Council Member of the African Association of Physiological Sciences, South Africa, and Council Member of the African Regional Training Network for Medical and Allied Health Sciences, South Africa.

Contents

Preface

Surgery entails breakage of the skin, which is a natural barrier to invasion by microorganisms, whether they are flora or attacking pathogens.

That being the case, surgical site infections occur when proper infection prevention measures are not adhered to.

Since many surgeries are performed continuously in many health care facilities all over the world, the occurrence and burden of surgical site infections constitute common problems for both patients and healthcare systems.

The outcomes of such infections for patients are limitless and can vary from length of time to heal to loss of life, with all that these entail.

Within the context of this book, surgical site infections will be discussed according to the most recent guidelines.

Manal Baddour
Professor of Microbiology and Immunology,
Faculty of Medicine,
Alexandria University,
Egypt

Section 1

Scope and Definitions

Chapter 1

Introductory Chapter: Surgical Site Infections - A Quick Glance

Manal Mohammad Baddour

1. Surgical site infections

Surgical site infections (SSIs) are infections of the incision or organ space that occur after surgery [1].

Thus, infections that occur in the wound created by an invasive surgical procedure are generally referred to as surgical site infections (SSIs). SSIs are one of the most important causes of healthcare-associated infections (HCAIs).

The United States Centers for Disease Control and Prevention (CDC) has developed a definition for SSI as an "infection related to an operative procedure that occurs at or near the surgical incision within 30 days of the procedure or within 90 days if prosthetic material is implanted at surgery." This CDC definition thus describes three levels of SSI [2]:

- *Superficial incisional*, affecting the skin and subcutaneous tissue. These infections might show localized signs such as redness, pain, heat, or swelling at the site of the incision or by the drainage of pus.

- *Deep incisional*, affecting the fascial and muscle layers. These infections can be detected by the presence of pus or an abscess, fever with tenderness of the wound, or a separation of the edges of the incision exposing the deeper tissues.

- *Organ or space infection*, which involves any part other than the incision that is opened or manipulated during the surgical procedure, for example, a joint or the peritoneum. These infections can be suspected by the drainage of pus or the formation of an abscess detected by histopathological or radiological examination or during re-operation.

The endogenous bacteria on a patient's skin are believed to be the main source of pathogens that contribute to surgical site infection [3]. To help prevent SSI, preoperative surgical site skin preparation standard of care entails scrubbing or applying alcohol-based preparations containing antiseptic agents prior to incision, most commonly chlorhexidine gluconate or iodine solutions. These agents have an excellent action against a wide range of bacteria, fungi, and viruses.

Assessment of risk factors for developing SSI can be generally grouped by patient, wound, and procedural variables.

Patient variables that increase risk of SSI include:

- Very young or very old age

- Diabetes

- Smoking

- Steroid use

- Immune compromised patients

- Colonized or infected remote body site

- Obesity

- Malnutrition

- Length of preoperative stay

- Wound contamination

Procedural variables that can affect the risk for SSI include factors related to preoperative skin preparation, sterilization protocols, and the surgery itself such as:

- Antimicrobial prophylaxis

- Duration of surgical scrub

- Preoperative hair removal

- Skin antisepsis protocol

- Choice of preoperative skin preparation

- Operating room ventilation

- Wound class

- Sterilization of instruments and environment

- Foreign matter in the surgical site

- Surgical techniques

- Duration of surgery

In 2016, the World Health Organization (WHO) published global guidelines for the prevention of surgical site infection which are evidence-based and present additional information in support of actions to improve practice [4].
Strong guideline recommendations by the WHO include:

- Patients with documented nasal carriage of *Staphylococcus aureus* should be decolonized by intranasal applications of mupirocin 2% ointment with or without chlorhexidine gluconate (CHG) body wash.

- Mechanical bowel preparation alone should NOT be used in adult patients undergoing elective colorectal surgery (without the administration of oral antibiotics).

- Hair should NOT be shaved whether before surgery or in the operating room. If absolutely necessary, hair should only be removed with a clipper.

- Preoperative antibiotic prophylaxis should be administered before surgical incision, when indicated.

- Preoperative antibiotic prophylaxis should be administered within 120 minutes before the surgical incision, taking into consideration the half-life of the antibiotic.

- Surgical hand preparation can be performed by either scrubbing with a suitable antimicrobial soap and water or by using a suitable alcohol-based handrub before donning sterile gloves.

- Alcohol-based antiseptic solutions based on CHG for surgical site skin preparation should be used in patients undergoing surgical procedures.

- Adult patients undergoing general anesthesia with endotracheal intubation for surgical procedures should receive 80% fraction of inspired oxygen intraoperatively and, if feasible, in the immediate postoperative period for 2–6 hours.

- Preoperative antibiotic prophylaxis administration should not continue after completion of the operation.

Actually, regarding a few of the WHO recommendations, the CDC stated that available evidence suggested uncertain trade-offs between the benefits and harms regarding such practices and that they advocated no recommendation/unresolved issue.

SSI rate is a percentage and is calculated as the number of SSIs divided by the total number of patients.

The rate of surgical site infections (SSIs) is low for most surgical procedures. However, because of the relatively large surgical volume in many hospitals, SSIs are sometimes considered the most common healthcare-associated infections [5]. SSIs are often localized to the incision site but can also extend into deeper adjacent structures [6].

Because of the presence of intraluminal bacteria, gastrointestinal procedures are among the highest risk procedures for SSI. Rates of SSI following bile duct, liver, or pancreatic surgery are as high as 10 per 100 procedures, according to data published by the National Healthcare Safety Network. Rates of SSI following colon surgery are ~5 per 100 procedures, and rates of SSI following gallbladder surgery are 0.7 per 100 procedures [7].

A prevalence survey undertaken in 2006 suggested that ~8% of patients in hospitals in the UK have a healthcare-associated infection (HCAI). SSIs accounted for 14% of these infections, and nearly 5% of patients who had undergone a surgical procedure were found to have developed an SSI. However, the true prevalence is expected to be higher since many of these infections occur after the patient has been discharged from hospital and are thus underreported and underestimated [8].

In an annual report from a UK hospital in 2009, the crude SSI rate was 4.4% [9].

Some studies done in Brazil, Sweden, China, and the USA report SSI prevalence rates of 7.2, 5.9, 6.2, and 2.9%, respectively, after appendectomy [10].

Within the context of this book, some of the risk factors and practices associated with SSI will be displayed, and an outline of the recommendations published by several authorities shall be portrayed. Additionally, since dental procedures pose a major concern in infection control, a comprehensive report on factors related to infection control in dentistry will be presented.

Author details

Manal Mohammad Baddour
Alexandria University, Alexandria, Egypt

*Address all correspondence to: manal.baddour@alexmed.edu.eg

IntechOpen

References

[1] National Healthcare Safety Network, Centers for Disease Control and Prevention. Surgical site infection (SSI) event. 2017. Available from: http://www.cdc.gov/nhsn/pdfs/pscmanual/9pscssicurrent.pdf [Accessed: 25 January 2017]

[2] Health Protection Agency. Surveillance of Surgical Site Infection in England: October 1997–September 2005. London: Health Protection Agency; 2006

[3] Mangram AJ, Horan TC, Pearson ML, Silver LC, Jarvis WR. Guideline for prevention of surgical site infection, 1999. Centers for Disease Control and Prevention (CDC) Hospital Infection Control Practices Advisory Committee. American Journal of Infection Control. 1999;27:97-132

[4] WHO global guidelines for the prevention of surgical site infection. 2016. Available from: https://www.who.int/gpsc/SSI-outline.pdf?ua=1

[5] Lewis SS, Moehring RW, Chen LF, et al. Assessing the relative burden of hospital-acquired infections in a network of community hospitals. Infection Control and Hospital Epidemiology. 2013;34:1229

[6] CDC/NHSN Protocol Corrections, Clarification, and Additions. April 2013. Available from: http://www.cdc.gov/nhsn/PDFs/pscManual/9pscSSIcurrent.pdf

[7] Edwards JR, Peterson KD, Mu Y, et al. National Healthcare Safety Network (NHSN) report: Data summary for 2006 through 2008, issued December 2009. American Journal of Infection Control. 2009;37:783

[8] National Collaborating Centre for Women's and Children's Health (UK). Surgical Site Infection, Prevention and Treatment of Surgical Site Infection. London: RCOG Press; 2008. NICE Clinical Guidelines, No. 74. ISBN-13: 978-1-904752-69-1

[9] Surgical Site Infection Surveillance (SSIS) for General Surgery. Wexford General Hospital Surgical Site Infection (SSI) data report; Annual report; 2009

[10] Rosenthal VD, Richtmann R, Singh S, et al. Surgical site infections, International Nosocomial Infection Control Consortium (INICC) report, data summary of 30 countries, 2005-2010. Infection Control and Hospital Epidemiology. 2013;34:597-604. DOI: 10.1086/670626

Chapter 2

Risk Factors and Key Principles for Prevention of Surgical Site Infections

Hadir Okasha

Abstract

Surgical site infections are one of the most important causes of healthcare-associated infections (HCAIs). They are associated with morbidity and possibly in part as a factor in associated postoperative mortality if present. Thus, it is important to recognize different SSIs and that they can vary from trivial wounds to a life-threatening condition. There are multiple risk factors contributing to the development of SSIs and guidelines to combat and decrease the possibility of the occurrence of such events through proper implementation.

Keywords: surgical site infections, hospital associated infections, criteria, classification, guidelines

1. Introduction

Infections occurring in the wound of an invasive surgical procedure are generally referred to as surgical site infections (SSIs), and they continue to be a common complication of surgical procedures despite advances in infection control practices.

This infection is a result of several factors that if combined would increase the risk of SSI together with the fact that the population is aging with longer average life expectancy meaning that not only the number of operations are likely to increase but also the SSI risk index for an aging population will be higher. Other clinical outcomes of SSIs include poor scars that are cosmetically unacceptable, such as those that are spreading, hypertrophic, or keloid; persistent pain and itching; and restriction of movement, particularly when over joints and have a significant impact on emotional well-being.

Given already the high economic cost of surgery, SSI will only burden the health system by increasing hospital stay, antibiotic intake, and other associated cost.

In this chapter we will briefly go through the pathogenesis and risk factors for SSI and guidelines to decrease their incidence.

2. Local events occurring on surgical incision

Most surgical wounds are contaminated by bacteria, yet infection will only develop in minority. As in the majority, innate host defenses will efficiently eliminate contaminants at the surgical site. This is besides other factors that interplay to give rise to a SSI including the inoculum of bacteria and its virulence and adjuvant microenvironment effects.

So what happens with the creation of the surgical incision through the skin and into subcutaneous tissues?

A. First, of course, there will be platelet and coagulation factor activation as part of hemostasis mechanisms, and this also marks the beginning of the inflammatory process.

B. Mast cells and complement proteins are activated, and bradykinin is produced from its precursors. The net effect of these factors is the production of non-specific chemoattractant signals and chemokine signals that "draw" variable leukocyte populations into the area of incision.

C. Also we get vasodilation and increased local blood flow at the site of the incision. Yet blood flow slows down in preparation for margination of phagocytes.

D. So we have increased vascular permeability and local vasodilation leading to edema fluid and increased space between endothelial cells, i.e., permeability, giving phagocytic access to the incised damaged tissue.

E. The increased vascular permeability provides phagocytic access to the injured soft tissue, while edema provides aqueous conduits for the navigation of these phagocytes through the normally condensed extracellular tissues.

F. Thus, this inflammatory process occurring at the site of injury is crucial for mobilization of phagocytes instantly into the incisional wound before significant intraoperative contamination occurs giving the patient an advantage against infection [1, 2].

3. Risk factors

Despite of efficient decontamination and antisepsis, bacteria may still enter the wound from the OR environment or instruments or surgical staff or from patients skin. The largest inoculum of bacteria was found to occur with operations involving a body structure heavily colonized by bacteria (bowel). Substantial numbers of bacteria are also present in the stomach of older patients who have hypo- or achlorhydria. Significant concentrations of bacteria are encountered in the biliary tract when patients are over 70 years of age or have obstructive jaundice, common bile duct stones, or acute cholecystitis [3]. Procedures involving the female genital tract will encounter 10^6–10^7 bacteria/mL. Procedures that enter into the oropharynx, lung, or urinary tract will have significant contaminants depending upon the duration and types of disease that are responsible for the operation. Notably, SSIs are generally the consequence of intraoperative contamination and seldom result from bacterial contamination from distant blood-borne seeding of the wound site during the postoperative period.

The larger the inoculum of bacterial contamination, the greater the probability of infection as the outcome. There are other factors that make a given bacterial inoculum to result in infection in a patient, while a similar inoculum of contamination in other patients has no such outcome. These are the local environment of the surgical site and the integrity of host defense of the patient. These factors include but not limited to surgical site hematoma, necrotic tissue from overuse of electrocautery, the presence of foreign bodies (e.g., sutures, particularly braided silk and other permanent braided suture materials) in the surgical site, dead space management, and manner of handling soft tissue and organs are all contributors to SSI. These are technical issues that are generally not covered in published guidelines but are of great significance in the prevention of infection [4].

Another determinant contributing to SSI is the virulence of the bacterial contaminant. The more virulent the bacterial contaminant, the greater the probability of infection. Coagulase-positive staphylococci require a smaller inoculum than the coagulase-negative species. Virulent strains of *Clostridium perfringens* or group A streptococci require only a small inoculum to cause severe necrotizing infection. *Bacteroides fragilis* and other Bacteroides species are ordinarily organisms of minimal virulence as solitary pathogens, but when combined with other oxygen-consuming organisms, they will result in microbial synergism and cause very significant infection following operations of the colon or female genital tract [5]. The virulence of the bacteria represents an intrinsic variable influenced by the surgery site and bacteria colonizing the patient and cannot easily be controlled by preventive strategies.

Another factor to consider is the integrity of host defenses as acquired impairment of host responses is objectively related to increased rates of SSI, as in the case of chronic illnesses, malnutrition, hyperglycemia, and conditions associated with prolonged intake of corticosteroids and other infection at locations remote from the surgical.

Thus it is important to collect data on different types of risk factors in order to analyze SSI outcomes, to identify high-risk patients, and to control for differences in the patient level risk; this is done through surveillance. Important data to be collected for all patients are at least age; sex; type of surgical procedure, whether elective or emergency surgery; the American Society of Anesthesiologists (ASA) score; timing and choice of antimicrobial prophylaxis; duration of the operation; and wound contamination class [6].

4. Important classifications

SSI can be classified according to the degree of microbiological contagion; this classification system is an adaptation of the American College of Surgeons wound classification scheme [7].

Wounds are divided into four classes:

Clean: An operative wound in which no infection and no inflammation is encountered, and the respiratory, alimentary, genital, or uninfected urinary tracts are not involved and are primarily closed.

Clean-contaminated: These are operative wounds that involve the respiratory, alimentary, genital, or urinary tracts but under controlled conditions and without unusual contamination. This category includes operations involving the biliary tract, vagina, appendix, and oropharynx.

Contaminated: These include, besides open, fresh, accidental wounds, operations with major breaks in sterile technique as in open cardiac massage or spillage from the gastrointestinal tract and incisions in acute inflamed tissues, including necrotic tissue without evidence of purulent drainage as dry gangrene.

Dirty or infected: This includes wounds with retained devitalized tissue and those with existing clinical infection or visceral perforation. In this group, it is suggested that the organisms causing postoperative infection were present in the operative field before the operation.

5. What are surgical site infection criteria?

According to the CDC [7], SSI is classified into:

1. Superficial

2. Deep

3. Organ/space

5.1 Superficial surgical site infection

Infection occurring within 30 days after any operative procedure and only the skin and subcutaneous tissue are involved must be associated with at least one of the following:

- Purulent drainage from the superficial incision, with or without culture testing

- Isolated organisms from an aseptically obtained specimen

- At least one of the following signs or symptoms: pain or tenderness, localized swelling, erythema, or heat and superficial incision deliberately opened by a surgeon

- Diagnosis of a superficial incisional SSI by the involved clinician

5.2 Deep incisional SSI

Infection involves deep soft tissues of the incision as fascial and muscle layers and occurs within 30 or 90 days after the operative procedure and must be associated with at least one of the following:

- Purulent drainage from the incision but not from the organ or space involved

- Isolated organisms from an aseptically obtained specimen

- Dehiscence or deliberate opening or aspiration by the surgeon from the deep incision when the patient has at least one of the following: fever greater than 100.4°F, localized pain, or edema, unless culture is negative

- An abscess or other evidence of infection involving the deep incision that is detected during anatomical or histopathologic exam or imaging

5.3 Organ/space SSI

It involves any part of the body deeper than the fascial/muscle layers, that is opened or manipulated during the operative procedure, and infection occurs within 30 or 90 days after the operation and must be associated with at least one of the following:

- Purulent drainage from a drain that is placed into the organ/space

- Organisms identified from fluid or tissue in the organ/space

- Abscess or other evidence of infection involving the deep incision that is found during examination of incision, reoperation, or pathologic or radiologic exam

6. SSI prevention guideline

A. In late 2016, the World Health Organization (WHO) provided guidelines offering ways to stop surgical infections including evidence-based recommendations, addressing the increasing burden of healthcare-associated infections on both patients and healthcare systems. They are suitable for any country and can be locally adapted [8].

B. In May 2017, the Centers for Disease Control and Prevention's (CDC) Healthcare Infection Control Practices Advisory Committee (HICPAC) published its Guideline for the Prevention of Surgical Site Infection, 2017, in the journal JAMA Surgery. Which also included evidence-based recommendations for the prevention of SSIs [9].

C. The Association of periOperative Registered Nurses (AORN) has published the 2018 Guidelines for Perioperative Practice with five updated guidelines, as well as a completely new guideline that addresses team communication. Guidelines for Perioperative Practice, published each January, is a collection of 32 guidelines that provide evidence-based recommendations to deliver safe perioperative patient care and achieve workplace safety. The AORN's Guidelines for Perioperative Practice is divided into five main topic areas: Aseptic Practice, Equipment and Product Safety, Patient and Work Safety, Patient Care, and Sterilization and Disinfection [10].

7. Key recommendations in guidelines

   i. Preoperative bathing

It is considered a good practice to advice patients to bathe or shower (full body) prior to surgery, with either plain soap or an antimicrobial soap on at least the night before the operative day.

   ii. For patients undergoing cardiothoracic and orthopedic surgery with known nasal carriage of *S. aureus*, decolonization with mupirocin 2% ointment with or without CHG body wash for the prevention infection in nasal carriers is recommended.

   iii. Administer preoperative surgical antibiotic prophylaxis (SAP) prior to the surgical incision when indicated (based on the type of operation, published clinical practice guidelines and while considering the half-life of the antibiotic, such that a bactericidal concentration of the agents is established in the serum and tissues when the incision is made). Topical antimicrobial agents should not be applied to the surgical incision.

   iv. As for postoperative antimicrobial prophylaxis in clean and clean-contaminated procedures, there is no need for additional antimicrobial prophylaxis doses after the surgical incision is closed in the operating room, even in the presence of a drain.

   v. Hair removal in patients undergoing any surgical procedure should either not be removed or, if necessary, should be removed with a clipper, since shaving is discouraged, whether preoperatively or in the OR.

vi. Performing surgical site skin preparation using an alcohol-based antiseptic solution is recommended unless contraindicated.

vii. Surgical hand preparation to be performed by scrubbing with either a suitable antimicrobial soap and water or using a suitable alcohol-based handrub before donning sterile gloves.

viii. Normothermia (i.e., a perioperative normal body temperature) to be maintained for all patients, in the OR and during the surgical procedure for reducing SSI.

However no randomized controlled trials evaluated methods to achieve and maintain normothermia and identified the lower limit of normothermia or the optimal timing and duration of normothermia for the prevention of SSI.

ix. Sterile drapes and gowns, either disposable or reusable woven drapes and gowns, must be used during surgical operations for the purpose of preventing SSI. On the other hand, the use of plastic adhesive incise drapes for preventing SSI was discouraged.

x. Wound protector devices were considered in clean-contaminated, contaminated, and dirty abdominal surgical procedures for the purpose of reducing the rate of SSI.

xi. Irrigation of incisional wound using saline before closure for preventing SSI was neither recommended for or against as no enough evidence were present for justification. However the use of an aqueous PVP-I solution for the irrigation of incisional wound before closure in clean and clean-contaminated wounds for the purpose of preventing SSI was recommended. While antibiotic incisional wound irrigation was recommended against, CDC considers intraoperative irrigation of deep or subcutaneous tissues with aqueous iodophor solution for the prevention of SSI but stated that for contaminated or dirty abdominal procedures, it is not necessary.

xii. Antimicrobial triclosan-coated sutures for the purpose of reducing the risk of SSI, independent of the type of surgery, were suggested.

xiii. Perioperative glycemic control implementation using blood glucose target levels less than 200 mg/dL in patients with and without diabetes is recommended.

xiv. Regarding postoperative phase, there are fewer recommendations identified across the guidelines in relation to wound care. For example, the WHO (2016) guidelines states: "The panel suggests not using any type of advanced dressing over a standard dressing on primarily closed surgical wounds for the purpose of preventing SSI."

xv. Team communication: AORN's Guidelines are the first evidence-based guideline to tackle the issue of effective communication in the perioperative environment which is essential for accurate transfer of patient information. The Editor in chief of AORN's Guidelines for Perioperative Practice stated that "Every AORN guideline recommends team involvement and shared communication with all stakeholders on the perioperative team, yet research still identifies ineffective team communication as a common cause of adverse events," and that "Understanding the evidence supporting strategies to strengthen team communication is critical for teams to successfully implement all AORN guidelines for safe perioperative care."

8. Surveillance

An effective infection prevention and control (IPC) program must not only apply measures and guidelines to avoid infections but should also monitor the outcome through surveillance. Which is defined as "the ongoing, systematic collection, analysis, interpretation and evaluation of health data closely integrated with the timely dissemination of these data to those who need it" [11].

9. Guideline implementation in reality

It is important that guidelines can be adapted with relative flexibility to suit different clinical situation in the context of availability of resources, training, and according to economic feasibility. Thus, the local situation in any institute would influence applicability and will therefore have a significant impact on implementing a certain guideline. Nonetheless, this does not negate the importance of having guidelines based on best evidence [12]. Rather, it emphasizes the extent to which evidence obtained in a specific setting is generally valid or applicable to other situations.

Thus implementation of evidence-based guidelines is a challenge in many healthcare settings, and it is not often easy to evaluate application and consistency of performance in clinical practice. It has been stated that it takes approximately 5 years for any given guidelines to be accepted and adopted into routine clinical practice and often not fully followed [12, 13]. This is because of the multifactorial nature of implementing these guidelines, where implementation is influenced by the patient, healthcare providers, institutional facilities, and management; yet implementation is meant to overcome these obstacles [13, 14].

That is why guidelines take relatively a long time to implement using different tools to bypass these problems, for example, not only vigorous and continuous education aiming to train individuals but also to change believes and misconceptions reflected on certain behaviors that have become second nature, especially if the recommendation requires infrastructure or a device that is not available or the practice opposes the cultural norms of a specific setting/group. Implementation tools that increase guideline acceptability and accessibility must use a variety of user-friendly formats directed to deliver the knowledge to all those involved in the issue including patients and different groups of HCWs among different settings [14]. Also as most of the suggested guidelines are not subjected to rigorous economic evaluation, it is important to keep this point in focus alongside with effectiveness during implementation, by using surveillance feedback which provide guidance to staff and decision-makers to lever support for the appropriate allocation of resources and efforts, helping clinicians in selecting the best available evidence-based options in healthcare organizations with limited resources.

Author details

Hadir Okasha
Medical Microbiology and Immunology, Faculty of Medicine, Alexandria
University, Egypt

*Address all correspondence to: shellm@gvsu.edu

IntechOpen

References

[1] Robson MC, Krizek TJ, Heggers JP. Biology of surgical infection. Current Problems in Surgery. 1973;**10**(3):1-62

[2] Heggers JP. Assessing and controlling wound infection. Clinics in Plastic Surgery. 2003;**30**:25-35

[3] Onderdonk AB, Bartlett JG, Louie T, et al. Microbial synergy in experimental intra-abdominal abscess. Infection and Immunity. 1976;**13**:22-26

[4] Fry DE. Prevention of infection at the surgical site. Surgical Infections. 2017;**18**(4). DOI: 10.1089/sur.2017.099

[5] Polk HC Jr, Miles AA. Enhancement of bacterial infection by ferric iron: Kinetics, mechanisms, and surgical significance. Surgery. 1971;**70**:71-77

[6] Protocol for Surgical Site Infection Surveillance with a Focus on Settings with Limited Resources. Geneva: World Health Organization; 2018. Licence: CC BY-NC-SA 3.0 IGO. https://www.who. int/infection-prevention/tools/surgical/ SSI-surveillance-protocol.pdf

[7] Centers for Disease control and prevention. Procedure-associated Module. SSI. Surgical Site Infection (SSI). Retrieved from: https://www.cdc.gov/nhsn/pdfs/ pscmanual/9pscssicurrent.pdf

[8] Global guidelines for the prevention of surgical site infection, second edition. Geneva: World Health Organization; 2018. Licence: CC BY-NC-SA 3.0 IGO. Retrieved from: https://www.medbox. org/preview/5c35b992-bb40-4beb-bcf0-1a3d1fcc7b87/doc.pdf

[9] Berríos-Torres SI et al. Centers for disease control and prevention guideline for the prevention of surgical site infection. JAMA Surgery (Published online May 3, 2017). 2017. DOI: 10.1001/ jamasurg.2017.0904

[10] Association of Perioperative Registered Nurses (AORN) Guidelines for Perioperative Practice, 2018 Edition: www.aornstandards.org/

[11] CDC/NHSN surveillance definitions for specific types of infections. Atlanta (GA): Centers for Disease Control and Prevention; 2017. Retrieved from https://www.cdc.gov/nhsn/pdfs/ pscmanual/17ps cnosinfdef_current.pdf

[12] Grol R, Grimshaw J. From best evidence to best practice: Effective implementation of change in patients' care. Lancet. 2003;**362**(9391):1225-1230. DOI: 10.1016/S0140-6736(03)14546-1

[13] Grimshaw J, Thomas RE, Maclennan G, Fraser C, Ramsay CR, Vale L, et al. Effectiveness and efficiency of guideline dissemination and implementation strategies. Health Technology Assessment. 2004;**8**(6):1-72

[14] Gagliardi AR, Brouwers MC. Do guidelines offer implementation advice to target users? A systematic review of guideline applicability. BMJ Open. 2015;**5**:e007047. DOI: 10.1136/ bmjopen-2014-007047

Section 2

Nursing Staff Contribution

Investigating the Factors Affecting the Hand Hygiene Compliance from the Viewpoints of Iranian Nurses Who Work in Intensive Care Units

Esmail Khodadadi

Abstract

Background: Hospital infections are known as one of the most important risk factors in healthcare units, and the hand hygiene is the first step in controlling these infections. Considering the importance of hand hygiene in reducing hospital infections, especially in intensive care units (ICUs), this study aimed to determine the factors affecting the compliance of hand hygiene among the ICU nurses in educational hospitals of Tabriz in Iran. Methods: This descriptive cross-sectional study was performed on 200 nurses working in ICU of educational hospitals in Tabriz. Sampling method determined the sample size and a 29-item researcher-made tool helped to collect data on demographic characteristics of nurses and organizational factors as self-report. The software SPSS 21 was used for descriptive analysis and statistics. Results: The results of this study showed that majority of nurses' viewpoint as an individual was affirmative by indicating: "positive effects of hand hygiene on reducing the incidence of hospital infections"; "skin irritation from repeated hand washes"; and "wearing gloves instead of using hygiene solution". The nurses' viewpoint on the organizational factors, distinguished: "working in ICU with simultaneous care of several patients"; "the type of hand washing solution used in the hospital"; "the availability of hand washing solutions at all times"; "the correct sink location"; "continuing education and retrain for ICU nurses"; "caring for isolated patients"; and "administrative support and their encouragement is effective for hand hygiene compliance". Conclusions: The results of this study showed that the level of hand hygiene compliance among the healthcare personnel who work in ICU, are associated with several personal and organizational factors. These results can facilitate institutional application of more effective hand hygiene procedures in ICU by specialized nurses and reduce the hospital infection rates.

Keywords: hand hygiene, personal and organizational factors, intensive care units, nurses

1. Introduction

Currently, the World Health Organization (WHO) has reported hospital infections as a serious global issue leading to prolonged hospitalization, ineffective treatments, increased costs, and high mortality [1, 2]. Hospital infections mostly occur in ICUs at 10–80% rates, and patients in these units are 5–7 times more likely to develop infections when compared to other units [3–5]. In fact, patients in the ICU units are more at risk for injuries due to the lack of full consciousness and weaker immunity [6, 7].

However, about 50% of hospital infections are caused by the hands of personnel [8]. Evidence suggests that wearing gloves reduces the risk of pathogen transmission to the patients by the healthcare staff. The World Health Organization has also emphasized the use of gloves when it comes to contact with body fluids and secretions or when necessary for meeting the precautionary requirements [1, 9]. In addition, studies have shown that hand hygiene role is not well known and an average of hand washings rate is usually less than 50% among nurses, so the majority of them wear gloves in order to protect themselves [6, 10, 11].

Other study findings show that healthcare personnel express various barriers for poor hand hygiene such as skin irritation, lack of hygiene products, negative view of patients when nurses wear gloves, forgetfulness, ignoring instructions, lack of time, high workload, personnel shortage, and lack of scientific evidence on hand hygiene reducing hospital infections [12–14]. On the other hand, evidence suggests that hand hygiene among the healthcare personnel is influenced by religion and culture [15]; attitude and awareness [16]; and personal and organizational factors [17]. The results of some studies have shown that personal factors such as age, gender, education, and the organizational factors include management style, work environment, and education are important factors among the healthcare personnel [17–19].

A review of the studies shows that the acceptance of hand hygiene among nurses is low [20, 21], and some studies have reported a direct correlation between hand hygiene rate among the nurses and medical staffs in ICU units and a statistical high rate of hospital infections [22–24]. Considering the importance of hand hygiene in reducing hospital infections, especially in ICUs, the review of previous studies show that the factors affecting the hand hygiene compliance on reduction of infection among hospitalized patients have not been explored among the Iranian ICU nurses; therefore, the present study aimed to investigate the factors affecting the compliance of hand hygiene among ICU nurses in several hospitals in Tabriz, Iran.

2. Materials and methods

This cross-sectional descriptive study was conducted in 2015, in Tabriz, Iran by targeting ICU nurses who worked in teaching hospitals. A total of 200 ICU nurses participated in this study by self-reporting a researcher-made 29-item questionnaire. There were two parts in the questionnaire for assessing nurses' demographic characteristics such as age, gender, and marital status. On the second part of the questionnaire, nurses were asked about personal (eight items) and organizational (21 items) factors. The scoring was based on the Likert scale from "very effective = 5" to "without effect = 1". The content validity of the questionnaire was established by several nursing professors from the Tabriz University of Medical Sciences. The reliability of the questionnaire was performed by a test-retest method, and the correlation coefficient of items was calculated to be 78%.

Information about the overall goals of the study was provided for all participants, and a written informed consent was signed by each participant. Voluntary participation and maximum confidentiality were emphasized. The informed consent and the study implementation were approved by the Ethics Committee of Tabriz University of Medical Sciences (No. 5/2079). The questionnaires were provided to ICU nurses, and completed questionnaires were collected. Descriptive statistics (percentage and frequency, mean, and standard deviation) were used to analyze the data using SPSS 21 statistical software.

3. Results

The demographic results of this study shown in **Table 1** consist of 200 ICU nurses from Tabriz hospitals in Iran. Majority of nurses were female, married, held an undergraduate degree, and their mean age was 33.9 ± 3.4. Most of them were working in various shifts and reported attending hand hygiene workshops.

Participating nurses agreed with the personal factors such as "positive effects of hand hygiene on reducing the incidence of hospital infections, hand injuries due to the use of washing solutions, high workload and lack of time, firm belief about the effect of hand washing, and wearing of gloves instead of hand hygiene" were effective factors in hands hygiene and identified items "mental disturbances, the preference of satisfying the patient's needs for hand hygiene, and the gender of nurses (male or female)" were ineffective or low for hands hygiene compliance (**Table 2**).

The findings of this study showed that majority of nurses had considered organizational factors including ICU employment, simultaneous care of several patients, type of hand washing solution, availability of hand washing solutions, presence and location of sinks in ICU, offering continuing education programs, emergency care for patients, care for isolated patients, and organizational support to be influential in hand washing behavior. Other organizational factors included short-term care such as vital signs control, sufficient amount of paper napkins, impacts of higher skill senior nurses on junior nurses, head nurse continuous

Demographic characteristics of nurses, N = 200		Number/percent
Gender	Female	135 (67.5)
	Male	65 (32.5)
Marital status	Married	129 (64.5)
	Single	71 (35.5)
Academic level	Bachelor's degree	173 (86.5)
	Master's degree	27 (13.5)
Work shift	Fix	47 (23.5)
	Circulate	153 (76.5)
Organizational position	Head nurse	16 (8)
	Practitioner	184 (92)
Hand hygiene educated experiences	Yes	141 (70.5)
	No	59 (29.5)
Age (year)	33.9 ± 3.4	
Work history (year)	9.38 ± 4.42	

Table 1.
Demographic characteristics of study participants.

No	Personal factors	Training effectiveness level: number (%)					
		Very effective	Effective	Somewhat effective	Little effective	Without effect	Mean
1	The positive effect of hand hygiene compliance on reducing the incidence of nosocomial infections	142 (71)	57 (28.5)	1 (5)	—	—	4.71
2	Skin damage due to the use of washing solutions	113 (56.5)	68 (34)	14 (7)	5 (2.5)	—	4.45
3	Prefer to meet patient's needs rather than hand hygiene	24 (12)	47 (23.5)	71 (35.5)	49 (24.5)	9 (4.5)	3.14
4	Workload and lack of time	33 (16.5)	114 (57)	34 (17)	13 (6.5)	6 (3)	3.78
5	Firm belief about effectiveness of hand washing	109 (54.5)	78 (39)	11 (5.5)	2 (1)	—	4.47
6	Preoccupation and negligence	12 (6)	27 (13.5)	61 (30.5)	91 (45.5)	9 (4.5)	2.71
7	Sex type of nurses	14 (7)	52 (26)	40 (20)	49 (24.5)	45 (22.5)	2.71
8	Sufficient wearing gloves instead of hand hygiene compliance	33 (16.5)	107 (53.5)	33 (16.5)	16 (8)	11 (5.5)	3.68

Table 2.
The influence of personal factors on hand hygiene compliance.

No	Organizational factors	Training effectiveness level: number (%)					
		Very effective	Effective	Somewhat effective	Little effective	Without effect	Mean
1	Being employed in ICU ward	84 (42)	76 (38)	28 (14)	11 (5.5)	1(.5)	4.16
2	Nonholiday work shifts	19 (9.5)	24 (12)	28 (14)	61 (30.5)	68 (34)	2.33
3	Holiday work shifts	15 (7.5)	25 (12.5)	30 (15)	63 (31.5)	67 (33.5)	2.29
4	Simultaneous care of a large number of patients	26 (13)	56 (28)	62 (31)	50 (25)	6 (3)	3.23
5	The need for prompt action in multiple care and procedures for several patients	19 (9.5)	8 (4)	59 (29.5)	101 (50.5)	13 (6.5)	3.73

No	Organizational factors	Training effectiveness level: number (%)					Mean
		Very effective	Effective	Somewhat effective	Little effective	Without effect	
6	Type of hand washing solution used in the hospital	95 (47.5)	69 (34.5)	21 (10.5)	11 (5.5)	4 (2)	4.20
7	Existence of sufficient amount of hand washing solutions	78 (39)	80 (40)	30 (15)	10 (5)	2 (1)	4.11
8	Existence of sufficient number of sink in ward	39 (19.5)	68 (34)	68 (34)	20 (10)	5 (2.5)	3.58
9	Putting sinks at the appropriate place in ward	38 (19)	46 (23)	90 (45)	22 (11)	4 (2)	3.46
10	Conducting continuing education programs (retraining) in the ward or hospital	27 (13.5)	60 (30)	82 (41)	29 (14.5)	2 (1)	3.41
11	Enough paper hold	43 (21.5)	33 (16.5)	80 (40)	35 (17.5)	9 (4.5)	3.33
12	Emergency care for critically ill patients	52 (26)	125 (62.5)	18 (9)	3 (1.5)	2 (1)	4.11
13	Caring for isolated patients	139 (69.5)	44 (22)	13 (6.5)	4 (2)	—	4.59
14	Carrying out short-term care such as blood pressure control	18 (9)	43 (21.5)	44 (22)	80 (40)	15 (7.5)	2.85
15	The impact of senior nurses "performance on novice nurses" performance	23 (11.5)	29 (14.5)	23 (11.5)	23 (11.5)	102 (51)	2.24
16	Continuous head nurse supervision for nursing staff	32 (16)	41 (20.5)	67 (33.5)	55 (27.5)	5 (2.5)	3.20
17	Give feedback about hand hygiene by the head nurse	28 (14)	42 (21)	68 (34)	58 (29)	4 (2)	3.16
18	Continuous supervision by infection control manager on nurses' hand hygiene	24 (12)	32 (16)	79 (39.5)	57 (28.5)	8 (4)	3.04
19	Give feedback about hand hygiene by infection control manager	26 (13)	29 (14.5)	79 (39.5)	58 (29)	8 (4)	3.04

No	Organizational factors	Training effectiveness level: number (%)					
		Very effective	Effective	Somewhat effective	Little effective	Without effect	Mean
20	Application of punitive methods by the organization's authorities	7 (3.5)	22 (11)	65 (32.5)	69 (34.5)	37 (18.5)	2.47
21	Applying encouragement methods by the organization's authorities	45 (22.5)	92 (46)	25 (12.5)	19 (9.5)	19 (9.5)	3.63

Table 3.
Effective organizational factors on hand hygiene compliance.

supervision on hand hygiene practice, getting feedback from infection control staffs, keeping organization's officials accountable in cases of "ineffective or low hand hygiene performance" (**Table 3**).

4. Discussion

The results of this study showed that several factors from nurses' point of view affected the hand hygiene practices. Based on their importance, these factors were attitude and beliefs about the impact of hand hygiene, the shortage of personnel and excessive workload, forgetfulness, and the belief in the cleansing solution hazards for the skin. In other studies, most nurses did not believe in hand hygiene, and the rate among medical personnel was low [12, 19, 21, 25, 26] pointing to a global concern [27]. Farbakhsh et al. found a low rate of hand hygiene practice among the Iranian nurses [28]. Similarly, Ghorbani et al. [29] showed that compliance of hand hygiene rate and wearing gloves among the nurses in ICU units was low, and most nurses used gloves without hand hygiene [29]. On the other hand, from the nurses' point of view, there were barriers to hand hygiene, which made it less likely for them to use hygiene while working with the patient. The results of Pan et al. research in 2013 revealed that hand washing could have negative effects on the skin, since frequent washing with soap resulted in dry skin, sensitivities, and dermatitis [30]. Therefore, nurses in certain places refrained from hand hygiene. In a study by De Wandel et al. [12], researchers found that disinfectant solutions with drying and irritation to the skin were obstacles to the hand hygiene practice. They reported that general attitude of nurses in ICUs were positive toward hand hygiene and increased work load did not directly affect health of their hands [12].

However, the results of other studies have indicated that a busy and high stressed environment negatively affect hand hygiene practices [31–33]. In a study by McArdle et al. [33], the shortage of personnel and heavy workload made hand hygiene less important because more time and energy were needed to take care of several patients [33]. High level of work pressure and nursing shortage generally affected the quality of nursing care [34–36]. Evidence suggests that knowledge and attitude of healthcare staff and how hand hygiene could reduce infection were directly influenced by the level of hands hygiene promotion [37–39]. In fact, the positive attitude of nurses showed that they were influenced by their knowledge about the scientific evidence of hand hygiene efficacy [16, 40]. Ravaghi et al.

[41] indicated that increased knowledge of personnel can improve their attitude toward hand hygiene. They also found that junior nurses were more accepting hand hygiene compared to senior nurses [41]. Nicol et al. [42] reported that staffs' sense of responsibility, work ethics, and level of experience played an important role on hand hygiene compliance [42]. While Whitby et al. [43] asserted that nurses had unpleasant feelings and discomfort regarding hand hygiene, where they had to be encouraged to protect themselves and ultimately change their attitude toward hand hygiene [43]. In contrast, Hazavehei et al. showed that personnel's level of knowledge and attitude toward hands hygiene was high, but these factors alone seemed insufficient to reach their goals [44].

In this study, we found that nurses in ICUs needed to enhance their hand hygiene practices. These results were inconsistent with findings of some researches in the past [14, 45, 46]. It is likely that different participants' attitudes and practices generated different results, and in this study, nurses' gender had no effect on the hand hygiene, while other studies indicated that female nurses practiced more hand hygiene than male nurses [19, 47]. Similar to this study, Nazari and Asgari found that hand hygiene practices were the same between male and female nurses [6].

Our findings, similar to other studies, showed that availability of hand sanitizer's increased the rate of hand hygiene among nurses and healthcare personnel, but heavy workload and overcrowding will reduce the rate [20, 31, 48]. Our findings of effective health education and staff encouragement on promotion of hand hygiene among the nurses were consistent with other study findings [49–52]. Ashraf et al. [31] showed that heavy workload and overcrowding limited hand hygiene, especially when there were insufficient supplies such as paper towels gloves, hand washing solutions, skin irritation due to persistent washing, and absence of washstand sink nearby [31]. Other studies have reported the lack of time and sinks [53], high workload, patient's condition, and lack of hand washing solutions [20], and lack of time as a reason for less hand hygiene practices [48]. In a review by Smiddy et al. [32], researchers showed that high workload and shortage of personnel were barriers to hand hygiene [32]. Other studies indicated that shortage of nursing staff in ICUs had a negative effect on hand hygiene and an increase in mortality rates [33]. In other words, a sufficient number of nursing personnel could effectively reduce the hospital infection rates [54] in support of the results of in this study.

5. Conclusions

Based on the results of present study, there are numerous personal and organizational factors affecting the compliance of hand hygiene among the ICU nurses. Working in ICU, personal beliefs, knowledge, and attitude toward the effects of hand hygiene on reducing infections; availability hand hygiene supplies; continuous health education training; and a supportive organizational management are all part of an effective hand hygiene practice. Therefore, these results could help hospital administrators to effectively implement policies to increase the rate of hand hygiene practices among the healthcare providers and hospital staffs to reduce preventable infections.

6. Limitations

The ICU nurses from Tabriz hospitals in Iran took part in this study, and researchers acknowledge the study limitation regarding generalizability of the results. Therefore, it is recommended that similar research to be conducted among a larger number of the ICU nurses in different cities to obtain an overall understanding of factors contributing to a low rate of hand hygiene.

Acknowledgements

Researchers are indebted to the officials at educational centers of hospitals in Tabriz for providing a research friendly environment. Our gratitude is also extended for the financial and spiritual support at the Nursing and Midwifery Faculty of Qazvin. We appreciate the participation of all ICU nurses in this research.

Author details

Esmail Khodadadi
PhD in Nursing Education, Iranian Social Security Organization, Iran

*Address all correspondence to: esmailkhodadadi11@gmail.com

IntechOpen

References

[1] Huis A, van Achterberg T, de Bruin M, Grol R, Schoonhoven L, Hulscher M. A systematic review of hand hygiene improvement strategies: A behavioural approach. Implementation Science. 2012;7:92

[2] Squires JE, Suh KN, Linklater S, Bruce N, Gartke K, Graham ID, et al. Improving physician hand hygiene compliance using behavioural theories: A study protocol. Implementation Science. 2013;8:16

[3] Amini M, Sanjary L, Vasei M, Alavi S. Frequency evaluation of the nosocomial infections and related factors in mostafa khomeini hospital ICU based on NNI system. JAUMS. 2009;7:9-14

[4] Mohammadimehr M, Feizabadi MM, Bahadori O, Motshaker arani M, Khosravi M. Study of prevalence of gram- negative bacteria caused nosocomial infections in ICU in Besat hospital in Tehran and detection of their antibiotic resistance pattern-year 2007. Iranian Journal of Medical Microbiology. 2009;3:47-54

[5] Vincent J-L, Rello J, Marshall J, Silva E, Anzueto A, Martin CD, et al. International study of the prevalence and outcomes of infection in intensive care units. JAMA. 2009;302:2323-2329

[6] Nazari R, Asgari P. Study of hand hygiene behavior among nurses in critical care units. Iranian Journal of Critical Care Nursing. 2011;4:95-98

[7] Rock C, Harris AD, Reich NG, Johnson JK, Thom KA. Is hand hygiene before putting on nonsterile gloves in the intensive care unit a waste of health care worker time?—A randomized controlled trial. American Journal of Infection Control. 2013;41:994-996

[8] Abdella NM, Tefera MA, Eredie AE, Landers TF, Malefia YD, Alene KA.

Hand hygiene compliance and associated factors among health care providers in Gondar University Hospital, Gondar, North West Ethiopia. BMC Public Health. 2014;14:96

[9] Loveday H, Lynam S, Singleton J, Wilson J. Clinical glove use: Healthcare workers' actions and perceptions. Journal of Hospital Infection. 2014;86:110-116

[10] Goldmann D, Larson E. Hand-washing and nosocomial infections. New England Journal of Medicine. 1992;327:120-122

[11] Jarvis W. Handwashing—the Semmelweis lesson forgotten? The Lancet. 1994;344:1311-1312

[12] De Wandel D, Maes L, Labeau S, Vereecken C, Blot S. Behavioral determinants of hand hygiene compliance in intensive care units. American Journal of Critical Care. 2010;19:230-239

[13] Larson E, Kretzer E. Compliance with handwashing and barrier precautions. Journal of Hospital Infection. 1995;30:88-106

[14] Pittet D. Improving adherence to hand hygiene practice: A multidisciplinary approach. Emerging Infectious Diseases. 2001;7:234

[15] Allegranzi B, Memish ZA, Donaldson L, Pittet D, Safety WHOGP. on Religious CTF, Religion and culture: Potential undercurrents influencing hand hygiene promotion in health care. American Journal of Infection Control. 2009;37:28-34

[16] Elaziz KA, Bakr IM. Assessment of knowledge, attitude and practice of hand washing among health care workers in Ain Shams University hospitals in Cairo. Journal of Preventive Medicine and Hygiene. 2009;50:19-25

[17] Larson EL, Early E, Cloonan P, Sugrue S, Parides M. An organizational climate intervention associated with increased handwashing and decreased nosocomial infections. Behavioral Medicine. 2000;**26**:14-22

[18] Lam BC, Lee J, Lau Y. Hand hygiene practices in a neonatal intensive care unit: A multimodal intervention and impact on nosocomial infection. Pediatrics. 2004;**114**:e565-e571

[19] van de Mortel T, Bourke R, McLoughlin J, Nonu M, Reis M. Gender influences handwashing rates in the critical care unit. American Journal of Infection Control. 2001;**29**:395-399

[20] Akyol AD. Hand hygiene among nurses in Turkey: Opinions and practices. Journal of Clinical Nursing. 2007;**16**:431-437

[21] Najafi Ghezeljeh T, Abbas Nejhad Z, Rafii F. A Literature Review of Hand Hygiene in Iran. Iran Journal of Nursing. 2013;**25**:1-13

[22] Bagheri P, Sepand M. The review systematic and meta analysis of prevalence and causes of nosocomial infection in Iran. Iranian Journal of Medical Microbiology. 2015;**8**:1-12

[23] Choi J, Kwak Y, Yoo H, Lee S-O, Kim H, Han S, et al. Trends in the incidence rate of device-associated infections in intensive care units after the establishment of the Korean Nosocomial Infections Surveillance System. Journal of Hospital Infection. 2015;**91**:28-34

[24] Dasgupta S, Das S, Chawan NS, Hazra A. Nosocomial infections in the intensive care unit: Incidence, risk factors, outcome and associated pathogens in a public tertiary teaching hospital of Eastern India. Indian journal of critical care medicine: Peer-reviewed, official publication of Indian Society of. Critical Care Medicine. 2015;**19**:14

[25] Albughbish M, Neisi A, Borvayeh H. Hand Hygiene Compliance among ICU Health Workers in Golestan Hospital in 2013. Jundishapur Scientific Medical Journal. 2016;**15**:355-362

[26] Shimokura G, Weber DJ, Miller WC, Wurtzel H, Alter MJ. Factors associated with personal protection equipment use and hand hygiene among hemodialysis staff. American Journal of Infection Control. 2006;**34**:100-107

[27] Erasmus V, Kuperus M, Richardus JH, Vos M, Oenema A, Van Beeck E. Improving hand hygiene behaviour of nurses using action planning: A pilot study in the intensive care unit and surgical ward. Journal of Hospital Infection. 2010;**76**:161-164

[28] Farbakhsh F, Shafieezadeh T, Zahraie M, Pezeshki Z, Hodaie P, Farnoosh F, et al. Hand Hygiene Compliance by the Health Care Staff in Medical centers affiliated to Shahid Beheshti Medical University. Tropical and Infectious Diseases Quarterly. 2013;**18**:9-13

[29] Ghorbani A, Sadeghi L, Shahrokhi A, Mohammadpour A, Addo M, Khodadadi E. Hand hygiene compliance before and after wearing gloves among intensive care unit nurses in Iran. American Journal of Infection Control. 2016;**44**:e279-e281

[30] Pan SC, Tien KL, Hung IC, Lin YJ, Sheng WH, Wang MJ, et al. Compliance of health care workers with hand hygiene practices: Independent advantages of overt and covert observers. PLoS One. 2013;**8**:e53746

[31] Ashraf MS, Hussain SW, Agarwal N, Ashraf S, Gabriel E-K, Hussain R, et al. Hand hygiene in long-term care facilities a multicenter study of knowledge, attitudes, practices, and barriers. Infection Control and Hospital Epidemiology. 2010;**31**:758-762

[32] Smiddy MP, O'Connell R, Creedon SA. Systematic qualitative literature review of health care workers' compliance with hand hygiene guidelines. American Journal of Infection Control. 2015;**43**:269-274

[33] McArdle F, Lee R, Gibb A, Walsh T. How much time is needed for hand hygiene in intensive care? A prospective trained observer study of rates of contact between healthcare workers and intensive care patients. Journal of Hospital Infection. 2006;**62**:304-310

[34] Aiken LH, Sloane DM, Bruyneel L, Van den Heede K, Sermeus W, Consortium RC. Nurses' reports of working conditions and hospital quality of care in 12 countries in Europe. International Journal of Nursing Studies. 2013;**50**:143-153

[35] Nantsupawat A, Srisuphan W, Kunaviktikul W, Wichaikhum OA, Aungsuroch Y, Aiken LH. Impact of nurse work environment and staffing on hospital nurse and quality of care in Thailand. Journal of Nursing Scholarship. 2011;**43**:426-432

[36] Van Bogaert P, Kowalski C, Weeks SM, Clarke SP. The relationship between nurse practice environment, nurse work characteristics, burnout and job outcome and quality of nursing care: A cross-sectional survey. International Journal of Nursing Studies. 2013;**50**:1667-1677

[37] Nair SS, Hanumantappa R, Hiremath SG, Siraj MA, Raghunath P. Knowledge, attitude, and practice of hand hygiene among medical and nursing students at a tertiary health care centre in Raichur, India. ISRN Preventive Medicine. 2014;1-4

[38] Pittet D, Simon A, Hugonnet S, Pessoa-Silva CL, Sauvan V, Perneger TV. Hand hygiene among physicians: Performance, beliefs, and perceptions.

Annals of Internal Medicine. 2004;**141**:1-8

[39] Sharif A, Arbabisarjou A, Balouchi A, Ahmadidarrehsima S, Kashani HH. Knowledge, attitude, and performance of nurses toward hand hygiene in hospitals. Global Journal of Health Science. 2016;**8**:57

[40] Nobile C, Montuori P, Diaco E, Villari P. Healthcare personnel and hand decontamination in intensive care units: Knowledge, attitudes, and behaviour in Italy. Journal of Hospital Infection. 2002;**51**:226-232

[41] Ravaghi H, Abdi Z, Heyrani A. Hand hygiene practice among healthcare workers in intensive care units: A qualitative study. Journal of Hospital. 2015;**13**:41-52

[42] Nicol PW, Watkins RE, Donovan RJ, Wynaden D, Cadwallader H. The power of vivid experience in hand hygiene compliance. Journal of Hospital Infection. 2009;**72**:36-42

[43] Whitby M, Pessoa-Silva C, McLaws M-L, Allegranzi B, Sax H, Larson E, et al. Behavioural considerations for hand hygiene practices: The basic building blocks. Journal of Hospital Infection. 2007;**65**:1-8

[44] Hazavehei MM, Noryan F, Rezapour Sahkolaee F, Moghimbayge A. Assessing the effective factors on hand hygiene using Planned Behavior Model among nursing and midwifery staff in Atea hospital of Hamadan in 2015. Journal of Hospital. 2016;**15**:51-58

[45] Pittet D, Boyce JM. Hand hygiene and patient care: Pursuing the Semmelweis legacy. The Lancet Infectious Diseases. 2001;**1**:9-20

[46] Samadipour E, Daneshmandi M, Salari M. Hand Hygiene Practice in Sabzevar hospitals Iran. Journal

of Sabzevar University of Medical Sciences. 2008;**15**:59-64

[47] Tai J, Mok E, Ching P, Seto W, Pittet D. Nurses and physicians' perceptions of the importance and impact of healthcare-associated infections and hand hygiene: A multi-center exploratory study in Hong Kong. Infection. 2009;**37**:320-333

[48] Kampf G, Löffler H, Gastmeier P. Hand hygiene for the prevention of nosocomial infections. Deutsches Ärzteblatt International. 2009;**106**:649

[49] Helder OK, Brug J, Looman CW, van Goudoever JB, Kornelisse RF. The impact of an education program on hand hygiene compliance and nosocomial infection incidence in an urban neonatal intensive care unit: An intervention study with before and after comparison. International Journal of Nursing Studies. 2010;**47**:1245-1252

[50] Picheansathian W, Pearson A, Suchaxaya P. The effectiveness of a promotion programme on hand hygiene compliance and nosocomial infections in a neonatal intensive care unit. International Journal of Nursing Practice. 2008;**14**:315-321

[51] Suchitra J, Devi NL. Impact of education on knowledge, attitudes and practices among various categories of health care workers on nosocomial infections. Indian Journal of Medical Microbiology. 2007;**25**:181

[52] Wisniewski MF, Kim S, Trick WE, Welbel SF, Weinstein RA, Project CAR. Effect of Education on Hand Hygiene Beliefs and Practices A 5-Year Program. Infection Control and Hospital Epidemiology. 2007;**28**:88-91

[53] Voss A, Widmer AF. No time for handwashing!? handwashing versus alcoholic Rub Can We afford 100% compliance? Infection Control and Hospital Epidemiology. 1997;**18**:205-208

[54] Hugonnet S, Harbarth S, Sax H, Duncan RA, Pittet D. Nursing resources: A major determinant of nosocomial infection? Current Opinion in Infectious Diseases. 2004;**17**:329-333

Section 3

Infections in Dentistry

Chapter 4

Infection Control in Dentistry and Drug-Resistant Infectious Agents: A Burning Issue. Part 1

Livia Barenghi, Alberto Barenghi
and Alberto Di Blasio

Abstract

Using molecular biological methods and retrospective investigations, some outbreaks in dental settings have been proven to be caused by mainly blood-borne viruses and water-borne bacteria. Nowadays, drug-resistant bacteria seem further hazards taking into account the worldwide overuse of antibiotics in dentistry, the limited awareness on infection prevention guidelines, and the lapses and errors during infection prevention (reported in more detail in Part 2). We chose MRSA and VRE as markers since they are considered prioritized bacteria according antibiotic resistance threats. Antibiotic-resistant bacterial infections inside of dental setting are relevant, and we argue about some hazards in dentistry, including dedicated surgeries. MRSA has a key role for its colonization in patients and dental workers, presence on gloves, resistance (days-months on dry inanimate surfaces), the contamination of different clinical contact surfaces in dental settings, the ability of some strains to produce biofilm, and finally its estimated low infective dose. For better dental patient and healthcare personnel safety, we need evidence-based guidelines to improve education and training initiatives in surgery.

Keywords: dentistry, surgery, guidelines, infection control, antibiotic resistance, biofilm

1. Introduction

Dentistry seems to provide safe procedures for oral health care taking into account all adverse events (AEs). Nevertheless, death, injury, and malfunctions due to dental devices (DDs) increased from the MAUDE report in 2000–2012, and the endosseous implants were at the top of the DDs involved in AEs [1]. In the same period, the number of malpractice payments in dentistry increased by 12%, while those in other health professions fell [2]. Dental AEs, complaints, and claims seem to be relatively common in different countries [3]. About 4–17% of AEs are due to infection [4, 5]. The iatrogenic infectious risk in dentistry has not been quantify closely yet [6, 7], but recently, some outbreaks caused by infective agents, mainly blood-borne viruses and water-borne bacteria, have been documented in dental settings based on molecular biological assays and/or retrospective investigations [8–11].

Some evidence exists around the hazard due of antibiotic-resistant infectious agents (ARIAs) in dentistry. Fatal adverse events (FAEs) had been reported within

90 days after different instances of dental care [7]. In the last 50 years, FAEs caused by an infection have (a) increased while respiratory complications and bleeding are steady, and those caused by cardiovascular or related to anesthesia have decreased, (b) significant (12%), (c) mainly associated to dental surgery (implant surgery/placement, extractions (>6 erupted teeth or impacted tooth/teeth), surgical extractions, osseous surgery, sinus lift surgery, bone biopsy, orthognathic surgery), and (d) associated with much longer times until death compared with other causes of death [7]. A study on dental malpractice analyzed 4149 legal claims (both in and out of court) from the years of 2000 to 2010 in Spain [12]. About 2.7% of all AEs resulted in death, and 45% of them were caused by infection. In the absence of specific information reported in both papers [7, 12], we do not exclude the possible involvement or nonrecognition of ARIAs or the failure of proper drug treatment in those FAEs. Recently, in an interview, Davies stated that in 20 years time even minor surgeries could be fatal because of infections [13].

We consider that the following two reviews are important and indicative of the limitedness of data published up to 2011–2012 in dentistry [14, 15]. The first review on methicillin-resistant *Staphylococcus aureus* (MRSA) infection concluded that (1) transmission was ascertained during surgical interventions, particularly in surgical units and among head and neck cancer patients; (2) carriage rates among dental healthcare personnel (DHCP) were lower than those among other health-care workers (HCWs); (3) carriage rates among adult patients were low, whereas among pedodontic and special care patients rates were higher than those found in the general population; and (4) MRSA had been detected in the environment of emergency, surgical units, and in dental hospitals [14]. In the second review, multi-resistant bacteria infections had been included among the main healthcare viral and bacterial infections in dentistry [15], but the transmission of Enterobacteriaceae and/or their resistant strains did not exist yet. The interest on Enterobacteriaceae is warranted since they are susceptible to only a few (if any) antibacterial drugs.

Here, we think it is important to update these conclusions in the light of the global, wide, and long-term abuse and misuse of antibiotics in dentistry and selective pressure on opportunistic bacteria by favoring potentially pathogenic strains [16, 17]. In addition, the limited awareness on infection prevention guidelines and lapses and errors during infection prevention according to Centers for Disease Control and Prevention (CDC) dental guidelines [6, 8–11] sustain the evidence of possible reservoirs of ARIAs in humans (patient, dental staff) and in the environment (clinical contact surfaces (CCSs), dental instruments, and dental unit water lines (DUWLs)) and possible hazards in surgical dental setting. Our approach is in line with the CDC recommendation, in which it states that *"Preventing infections negates the need for antibiotic use in the first place, and scientific evidence shows that reducing antibiotic use in a single facility can reduce resistance in that facility"* [18–20].

In addition, the cluster of above problems is important for risk management, since it is rationally "harmful" that opportunistic species and/or ARIAs were involved in implant failures [21, 22], periodontitis [23, 24], endodontic failures [25] and oral mucosal and deep infections [26].

Here, we discuss briefly main recent evidence and controversy on infections in dedicated dental and mainly in implant surgery, taking into account that many other aspects (i.e. surgery technique, geometry, materials, and surface of dental implants) have already been reviewed extensively [27–30]. Dental implant (DI) complications are a burning issue, since the current demand of DIs is high (20 DIs in Italy and 4 in the USA per year per million of inhabitants), mainly applied in private offices, and the global DI market size was estimated at 3.77 billion USD in 2016 growing at a compound annual growth rate (CAGR) of 7.7% over 2024 [31]. It is important to underline that the incidence of esthetic, technical and infective complications is still high in implantology, and the 5-year infective complication increased from 7.4 to

9.4% [32]. In general, the expected implant-associated infections and the outbreaks from opportunistic pathogens (*Staphylococci, Enterococci, Pseudomonas,* etc.) will always be more important. In addition, we have to take into account other factors linked to risk management such as the impact on reputation and finances, the loss of protection of insurance coverings and reimbursements, and shocking advertising rapidly spreading through social networks in the case of outbreaks [8–11, 33–35].

Here (Part 1), we focus on the insufficient compliance with infection control (IC) recommendations in oral healthcare and the difficulties and problems of standard precaution implementation also in ambulatory surgical centers [6, 36–42]. In general, dental surgery and implantology are predominantly done in general dental practice under local anesthesia or sedation [43, 44]. This is a very important aspect since the cross-infection is widespread and more difficult to control compared to surgical rooms. We have divided problems and difficulties for infection prevention into different areas concerning the innovative molecular biology techniques; antibiotic misuse and overuse in dentistry; opportunistic pathogens and antibiotic resistance in dental patients and dental healthcare workers; and surgical infection prevention in dentistry. While in the chapter (Part 2), we have reported infection control implementation, not compliance, lapses and errors during infection prevention according to CDC dental guidelines. We focused on hand hygiene, gloves, environment decontamination, and instrument reconditioning in more detail [6, 43–47].

2. Approach

The electronic literature search was conducted via the PubMed and Google Scholar databases (from January 2010 up to and including April 2018) using various combinations of the following key indexing terms: (a) patient safety; (b) infection control; (c) implant; (d) endodontia; (e) sterilization; (f) reconditioning; (g) critical items; (h) semicritical items; (i) hand hygiene; (j) DUWL; (k) sharps safety; (l) personal protective equipment (PPE); (m) disinfection; (n) MRSA; (o) VRE; (p) ARIAs; (q) guidelines; and (r) cross-infection. In addition, manual searches were carried out in INTECH books. Then, bibliographic material from the papers has been used in order to find other or older appropriate sources. A total of 179 papers and links were found suitable for inclusion in this chapter (Part 1). Only few papers do not have a DOI or PubMed classification, but the available link by Internet and accessed date have been added.

3. Focus on molecular biology techniques

Expanded Human Oral Microbiome Database (eHOMD) provides the scientific community with broad and up-to-date information on the bacterial species present in the human aero-digestive tract, including the oral cavity. Genomes for 482 taxa (63% of all taxa, 89% of cultivated taxa) are currently available on eHOMD [48]. Fast and very sensitive molecular biological techniques, classified into nucleic acid-based methods [quantitative real-time polymerase chain reaction (PCR), multiplex PCR, microarray, next-generation sequencing technologies, etc.], are available for the screening, detection, and functional activities of pathogens and antibiotic-resistant bacteria, even those not cultivable by classical microbiological methods and by using both patient biological fluids and samples from inanimate objects (surface, air, DUWL colonization, DDs, and instruments) [49–52]. This is possible because DNA molecules can survive for long time and can be amplified. Current microbiological laboratory approaches based on high-throughput real-time

PCR allow quick, easy, and cheap detection of the oral microbiome and the antibiotic resistome, throughout 300 antibiotic resistance genes [53] as far as the rapid diagnosis of virulent slime-producing strains associated with dental caries [54]. The specificity of MRSA plus MSSA carriage detected with Xpert MRSA is better than standard culturing techniques, being 37.9 vs. 23.6%, respectively [55]. Concerning microbiological features of peri-implantitis cases, culture methods were able to detect 81.4% of the targeted species of the cases, whereas "checkerboard DNA–DNA hybridization" method 99.3%. In relation to the limited association between the bacterial contamination and the severity of the peri-implantitis [56], it is decisive the sampling procedure, around DIs and during swabs on dental items, and the use of the proper primer sequence for specific genes in different strains (i.e. ica genes for *S. epidermidis and S. aureus*) [57]. PCR is more effective in detecting *E. faecalis* than other analytical tools, such as culturing. *E. faecalis* has been found in root-filled teeth associated with periradicular lesions in a range of 0–70% by culture and 0–90% by PCR [58].

It is important to note that microbiological analysis (by culture or DNA-based methods) is rarely used in dentistry mainly because of the difficulties to delay the antibiotic treatment and for the plethora of infective agents involved in inflammatory diseases in dentistry. In addition, specific sampling procedures are needed since the virulence features of microorganisms and problems to sample deep periodontal and peri-implant pocket and abscesses. Sequencing methods that evaluate the entire microbiome are needed to improve identification of microorganisms (pathogen, opportunistic, noncultivable, drug-resistant ones) associated to peri-implant infective diseases and to develop suitable countermeasures with the expertise of clinical oral microbiologists [59]. In addition, emerging approach based on optical nanoprobes, biosensors, and protein biomarkers suitable for peri-implant crevicular fluids has been proposed to identify the severity and progression of the disease and the response to therapy [60, 61].

4. The broad antibiotic misuse or overuse in dentistry

Globally, antibiotic prescription in dental care has continuously increased over the last 17 years, and a lot of evidence has been published on wide antibiotic misuse or overuse, in industrialized, low- and middle-income countries [62–70]. Dental prescriptions make up 5–11% of all antibiotic prescription among patients in some European countries, Canada, and the USA [19, 20, 65, 71, 72]. The rate of prescription increased the most among dental patients of 60 years or above.

It is important to underline that antibiotic prescription is placed without a microbiological analysis and has mainly prophylactic aim in dentistry. Recently, the prescription of antibiotics in dentistry was reviewed by Holmstrup and Klausen, while the use of antibiotics in odontogenic infections, in addition to the removal of the source of infection, by Martins [73, 74]. A significant percentage (19–37.5%) of microorganisms collected from their patients were penicillin resistant; nevertheless, the relationship between the clinical outcomes and microbial resistance with penicillin is not clear [74].

Recently, to overcome the misuse and abuse of antibiotics in dentistry, different institutions and associations recommended a more restrictive antibiotic policy to improve treatment efficacy and decrease bacterial resistance. Specific guidelines have been published for implantology [17], endodontia [75], oral surgery [17], third molar extraction [76], and medically compromised patients [77] and to prevent infective endocarditis [78, 79] or prosthetic joint infections [80].

5. Focus on opportunistic pathogens and antibiotic resistance in dental patients and dental healthcare workers

Here, based on recent and current knowledge, we focus on two well-known bacterial strains, *S. aureus* and *Enterococcus*, and their resistant strains. It is known that *S. aureus* and *Enterococcus faecalis* have been implicated in implant-associated infections [21, 23, 24, 81], endodontic infections [22, 25, 82], and recently in an outbreak of *Enterococcus* endocarditis [11]. We focus on these Gram-positive bacteria for the high innate resistance or ability to become resistant to most antibiotics along with some other virulence factors (hydrophobicity, adherence to abiotic surfaces (including dental implant materials), biofilm formation, ability to growth also in anaerobic conditions) [83]. These features are important in the exploration of standard precaution failures since bacterial adherence on dental implants, collagen-based biomaterials, or many other inanimate objects is known to be linked with the presence of surface components with nonpolar/hydrophobic vs. polar/hydrophilic characteristics. In addition, we focus on Staphylococci and Enterobacteriaceae as markers since they are considered prioritized bacteria according to antibiotic resistance threats, and better knowledge is available on their virulence factors and for dental settings (i.e. contamination on hands and environments, etc.) [6, 43, 45–47].

5.1 *Staphylococcus aureus* and MRSA

Single dose of prophylactic antibiotics in healthy volunteers induces a significant selection of resistant strains among the dynamic and complex community of resident oral and gastrointestinal bacterial microflora and causes a large disturbance of oral niches [84, 85]. Approximately, one third of participants gained resistant viridans *Streptococci* against amoxicillin, clindamycin, and penicillin-V, while in *Prevotella* spp., there was approximately a 28% gain in resistance to all antibiotics tested. The disturbance could reduce host colonization resistance, select new pathogens, and lead to an overgrowth of resistant bacteria [86].

S. aureus lives as a commensal primarily in the anterior nares and/or throat of 20–70% of adults [87, 88]. Some of the strains develop multidrug resistance and are well known to be involved in hospital-acquired (HA) infections [89]. The following two reviews are important and indicative of the limitedness of data published up to 2011–2012 in dentistry [14, 15]. *S. aureus* was normally absent or its colonization was very low in oral biofilm and ecological oral niches as reported in older evidence or not considered as a topic [14, 43, 90]. More recent data show that the presence of *S. aureus* in the oral cavity is more frequent and, nowadays, is to be considered a member of the oral microbiota (**Table 1**) [15, 84, 91–105]. Recently, metaproteomic analysis of human salivary supernatant from healthy persons was able to identify peptides from 124 microbial species including *Staphylococcus* [85]. The majority of *S. aureus* strains, isolated from the oral cavity of Tunisian patients, were biofilm/slime producers and exhibited some important genes (i.e. *ica, fnb, cna*) associated to adhesion and virulence factors [106, 107]. *S. pneumoniae* and *S. aureus* are common commensals of the upper respiratory tract in children and adolescents [14, 100, 108]. This fact is relevant since orthodontic patients are mainly children and adolescents and the high genotypic expression of peculiar genes (*ica*A/*ica*D) is important for *S. aureus* in the colonization of orthodontic appliances [109]. Recently, RNA-Seq data permit the analysis of active transcripts, assigned to antibiotics and toxic compounds, of the
supragingival dental plaque biofilm in healthy subjects [110]. The transcripts assigned to Acriflavin resistance complex (*AcrA* and *AcrB* genes) were prevalent,

Study	References	Study population	Number of subjects	Study carried out (years):	Country	Sampling, specimen, assay	*S. aureus* carriage (%)	MSSA carriage (%)	MRSA carriage (%)
Roberts et al. (2011)	[91]	Dental students	61	#	USA	Swab, anterior nose; §	#	21	21.3
Martinez-Ruz et al. (2014)	[92]	Dental students	100	#	Mexico	Paired nasal and throat swabs; §	#	#	20
Petti et al. (2015)	[93]	Dental students	157	#	Italy	Dry cotton swabs from the mouth, nose, and skin between fingers of the nondominant hand; §	15.3 (9.7–20.9), any site	#	0, any site
Baek et al. (2016)	[94]	Dental students	159	#	Korea	Nasal samples; §	#	#	3.1
Hema et al. (2017)	[95]	Dental students	200	#	India	Swab, anterior nares; §	#	#	24.5
Zimmerli et al. (2009)	[96]	500 dental patients >18 years	500	2006	Switzerland	Swab, anterior nares; §	42	41.6	0.4
McCormack et al. (2015)	[97]	10-year retrospective analysis of laboratory data	1429	1998–2007	UK	Perioral clinical specimens (no. 1986); §		90	10
Kabanova et al. (2017)	[98]	Patients from 5 maxillofacial departments	2920	2014	Belarus	Swabbing the area after the incision (no. 162); §	15–70	#	5.6–27.8
Dulon et al. (2014), review	[99]	HCW in non-outbreak settings	21,289 subjects from 31 studies	#	#		#	#	1.1–5.4 from high quality studies

Study	References	Study population	Number of subjects	Study carried out (years):	Country	Sampling, specimen, assay	S. aureus carriage (%)	MSSA carriage (%)	MRSA carriage (%)
Esposito et al. (2015)	[100]	Healthy subjects aged 6–17 years	497	2013	Italy	Oropharyngeal and nasal swabs; multiplex real-time PCR	#	49.7 from 6–9 years.; 54.9 from 10–14 years.; 52.9 from 15–17 years	3.5 (15–17 years)
Koukos et al. (2015)	[101]	Healthy patients	154	2010–2014	Greece	Subgingival samples and PCR assay	10	#	0
Kharialla et al. (2017)	[102]	Patient and DHCP	#	2013	Egypt	Swab, anterior nares, (no. 1300); culture plus molecular typing	8.6	#	11.1 patients; 6.7 nurses; 9.3 dentists
Yoo et al. (2018)	[103]	DHCP	139		Korea	Swab, anterior nares; §	#	#	2.9

§: using microbiological culture methods; PCR: polymerase chain reaction; #: not indicated.

Table 1.
Staphylococcus aureus, methicillin-sensitive Staphylococcus aureus (MSSA), and methicillin-resistant Staphylococcus aureus (MRSA) carriage rates among dental students, dental patients, dental healthcare personnel (DHCP), and healthcare workers (HCWs).

while those encoding for putative macrolide-specific efflux system or proteins involved in acid stress and bacteriocins are less represented. High percentages of *Staphylococcus* species, MRSA, *P. aeruginosa*, and *C. albicans* were detected in the mouths of elderly patients [111, 112]. By PCR, a notable occurrence of MRSA, vancomycin-resistant *S. aureus* (VRSA), and VSSA have been observed in the oral cavity of patients with dental caries [113]. Chronic periodontitis showed extensive antibiotic-resistant subgingival periodontal pathogens in cultivable microbiota, associated with red and orange complex species, and also to Gram-negative enteric rods/Pseudomonads, *E. faecalis*, and *S. aureus* [21, 23, 24, 114].

Here, we report updated data on *S. aureus* and MRSA carriage rates among dental students, dental patients, HCWs, and dental healthcare personnel (DHCP) in **Table 1** [91–103]. Despite the many differences between studies, nowadays there is a probable occupational exposure, from carriage rates, among DHCP and HCWs. This is higher in dental students (**Table 1**), but would seem evident in the last years [14, 91–95]. Nasal MRSA colonization, confirmed by the presence of the *mecA* gene that encodes a low-affinity penicillin-binding protein, occurs in dental students (3.1%), especially those who have clinical experience [94]. MRSA hand and nasal carriage rates in patients, nurses, and dentist are significant in dental settings (**Table 1**) [102]. The majority of MRSA isolates were multidrug resistant, and full resistance was generally higher for personnel than for the environmental isolates.

5.1.1 Community- and hospital-acquired MRSA infections and dentistry

Taking into account MRSA carriage in dental patients and DHCP, the effectiveness of MRSA decolonization, and the violation of IC precautions (see below and in Part 2), MRSA in the oral cavity could potentially be disseminated by carriers (patient and DHCP) to the environment [115]. It is well known that community-acquired MRSA (CA-MRSA) infections often occur in young and healthy individuals, whereas HA-MRSA infections occur predominantly in elder or immunocompromised patients in healthcare settings and vary considerably between different countries [116, 117].

HA-MRSA and CA-MRSA have opposite features concerning competitive fitness, virulence, and antimicrobial resistance [118]. Only rarely HA-MRSAs cause infections in healthy subjects, but at least two CA-MRSAs (USA300 and ST30) cause HA infections. It is not known if these strains acquire multiple resistant genes from HA-MRSA or if they increase bacterial fitness and survival despite the antibiotic resistance. Taking into account that their extracellular proteome seems to be differently involved, we think that this epidemiological change is not soothing for future dental epidemiology. In fact, from a 10-year retrospective analysis of laboratory data, obtained from oral and perioral clinical specimens, most of the MRSA isolates were epidemic MRSA-15 (EMRSA-15) or EMRSA-16 lineage, known to cause both very dangerous HA-MRSA infections [97]. No MRSA isolates belonging to community-acquired recognized lineages were identified. An alarming genetic similarity has been shown between seven MRSAs isolated in dental clinic and the EMRSA-15 clone [102]. In addition, *S. aureus*, MSSA, and EMRSA-15 harbored differently on dentures of in- and outpatients [119].

5.2 *Enterococcus faecalis*

It is well known that antibiotic administration causes intestinal overgrowth of *Enterococci* and their translocation across a histologically normal intestinal epithelium; then, they can reach and avidly bind other soft tissues and endocardial tissue matrix components, causing infections, abscess, and endocarditis. There are some reasons to consider *Enterococci* important for our topic. *E. faecalis* occurs in transient opportunistic infections involving the oral cavity and has been found in common dental diseases (i.e. caries, endodontic infections, periodontitis) and peri-implant infective disease, and its strains are peculiar in comparison to food ones [120]. Recently, public health officials reported an incidence rate of enterococcal endocarditis among the total patient population at the oral surgery practice, more than 200 times the expected rate among general population [11].

In addition, *E. faecalis* is so invasive that it is used to test dental materials (composite fillings, endodontic sealers, etc.) and the connection between DI and the abutment [121]. Since it is highly adhesive, has many virulence factors (resistance to extreme conditions (oxygen tension, pH, salts), collagen-binding proteins, gelatinase E, surface proteins), and the ability to form biofilm, *E. faecalis* can reside widely in and around tooth root canals, in the surrounding bone trabeculae, and in heavily infected subgingival sites [122, 123]. It is known that *E. faecalis* resistance to antibiotics has been increasing over time. Then, the oral cavity can constitute a reservoir for virulent E. faecalis strains possessing antibiotic resistance traits, able to transfer vanA resistance genes to MRSA [102] and with biofilm formation capabilities. The latter facilitates the exchange of genetic material (via horizontal gene transfer) important for resistance acquisition [120]. Tetracycline, erythromycin, clindamycin, and metronidazole revealed poor levels of *in vitro* activity against human subgingival *E. faecalis* clinical isolates [122].

Nowadays, Enterobacteriaceae and some resistant strains are present in oral cavity of dental patients, and recently, the transmission in dental practice has been proven [11, 120–124]. For dentistry of the future, whole-genome sequencing seems promising to study *Enterobacteriaceae* antimicrobial resistance based on genotype alone [125] and the role in dental implant-associated infections.

6. Surgical infection prevention in dentistry: from gold standard to reality

It is well known that the best choices for dental and implant surgery are a specialized and well-trained dental staff (surgeon, clean nurse, second nurse, anesthetist, etc.) and a specific designed surgical room with proper isolation, clean air system ventilation, instruments for automatic surface decontamination and ISO standards (UNI EN ISO 14644-ISO 5) that allow a very low environmental contamination, and proper antiseptic procedures (including hand washing, wearing, safe instruments passages). Unfortunately, this setting up is used in the case of maxillofacial surgery, and it is commonly present and economically sustainable in hospital surgical dental department. In ambulatory dental offices, there is no isolation and a full separation of the environments used for general dentistry and those used for implant surgery or dental extractions. Only rarely is present a clean air ventilation system according to ISO standards. This difference is very important since in general dental practices the cross-infection is widespread, and the infection prevention is more difficult or less controllable (i.e. absence of the second nurse, environmental contamination) compared to hospital surgical rooms. There are few controls legislated over the operating environment in ambulatory and private dental offices.

Bearing in mind the higher risk of contamination of ambulatory surgical areas, above all during long surgeries (sinus lift, several implant placing, guided bone regeneration (GBR)) and in medically compromised patients, we cannot exclude that a part of implant failures is the result of a chain of personnel latent errors, including some improper antiseptic measures (not surgical hand hygiene, unsterile gloves, improper use of mask, contamination of operating surface or room air, unsterile barrier covering, lack of surgical guide disinfection and mouth rinses, suture contamination by perioral skin bacteria, among others), as far as untrained professional practice [17, 41, 42, 44, 126].

Maintaining sterile conditions during the surgical procedure is of utmost importance. Saliva, perioral skin, unsterile instruments, contaminated gloves, operating room air, or air expired by the patient, all interfere in the surgical procedure leading to contamination of the implant site [43, 45–47]. It has been reported that the prevalence rate of MRSA was the highest in samples from dental surgery compared to other dental environments [102]. MRSA's involvement in surgical infections is in line with the estimated infective dose, which is very low (4 CFU), and surface contamination (<10 CFU/cm^2) [127, 128]. In ambulatory surgical centers, the main infection control lapses identified were hand hygiene and use of PPE, injection safety and medication handling, equipment reprocessing, and environmental cleaning [41, 42, 129].

The majority of DIs are predominantly placed in general dental practice under local anesthesia. Concerning local anesthesia, hand contact is the main source of the wide contamination reported on anesthetic syringes and anesthetic tubes used in dentistry [130]. Then, DHCP has to follow scrupulously key recommendations for safe injection reported in CDC guidelines [6]. Taking into account the recent outbreaks, the violations seem very hazardous in dentistry [8, 11]. In addition, it is absolutely forbidden and highly risky in the reuse of whatsoever single use sterile medical devices (i.e. irrigation sets) and the use of the water from DUWLs during implant and piezoelectric surgery, etc. [6]. The use of sterile devices and instruments is a need during surgical cares, but even after reconditioning, the contamination of surgical dental instruments and drills is significant even in hospital settings [131–134]. Many other specific failures concerning dental instrument reconditioning will be discussed in Part 2. The importance of hand hygiene, sterile gloves, mask, and eye protection during surgery is well known. Violations are frequent and often surgical videos in dentistry show the surgical mask *under the nose,* that is risky taking into account MRSA nose colonization in dentists and dental nurses. We underline that it is a hazard to touch the barrier membranes during GBR with gloved hands: this is a frequent slip observed in untrained surgeons.

6.1 Infections associated to craniofacial skeleton

The most relevant infections are lateral and apical periodontitis, osteomyelitis, peri-implantitis, and their complications, such as facial cellulitis and other infections involving deep spaces of face and neck [135]. Microbiota associated with infections of the craniofacial skeleton, particularly maxilla and mandible, are polymicrobial in nature and a mix of aerobic-anaerobic genera. In head and neck space odontogenic infections, the most common bacteria isolated were Gram-positive cocci (*Viridans streptococci, Prevotella, Staphylococci, and Peptostreptococcus*), and discordant data have been reported on antibiotic resistance of *Viridans streptococci,* while very few isolates of *Staphylococcus* are now susceptible to penicillin [136, 137].

Taking into account the increasing life expectancy, it is important to underline that older patients, even without systemic diseases, are more prone to development of oral pathology infections because of often lower immunological response [138]. Concerning systemic and local odontogenic infection complications requiring hospital care, an analysis showed that medically compromised patients appear more susceptible to systemic rather than local infection complications with a need for significantly longer hospital stay and with an increased risk for fatal complications [139].

The main causative agents of maxillofacial inflammatory diseases are *S. aureus*, *S. epidermidis*, *Streptococcus* spp., *Escherichia coli*, and *Proteus* spp. [85]. Concerning the risk of maxillofacial surgeries, 4% of their patients showed odontogenic infections, and about 2–20% required intensive medical therapy after surgery [140, 141]. These compliances are expected to worse taking into account the current oral carriage of *S. aureus* and MRSA (**Table 1**) and the presence of epidemic MRSA-15 (EMRSA-15) or EMRSA-16 lineage in dental settings.

Results have been conflicting concerning the occurrence of bacteremia after dental procedures; antimicrobial prophylaxis before an invasive dental procedure does not prevent bacteremia, although it can decrease both its magnitude and its persistence [142]. Delayed-onset infections (DOI) after mandibular third molar extractions are rare complications and usually occur about 30 days after the extraction, but they may also develop much later on [143]. The bacteria identified in DOI are *Fusobacterium*, *Prevotella*, *Bacteroides*, and *Peptostreptococcus*. A recent review reported in detail several oral and maxillofacial fungal infections, including mucormycosis, candidiasis, aspergillosis, blastomycosis, histoplasmosis, cryptococcosis, and coccidioidomycosis [144].

6.2 Infective agents in dental implantology

In general, dental implant procedures are considered clean-contaminated surgeries (graded as class II surgical procedures), since micro-organisms living in the oral mucosa and in saliva contaminate the surgical wound facilitating the infection, with local infection rates of 10–15% and an incidence of infection to 1% or less by the use of both prophylactic antibiotics and proper surgical technique [71]. Despite the statements reported between 1980 and 1990, even in the case of the use of prophylactic antibiotics, the reported prevalence of postoperative infection after implant installation ranges from 0 up to 11.5% and the prevalence of peri-implantitis varied from 4.2 to 47% of all implants [21, 56, 69, 71, 84, 114, 145–149]. These data are higher than the annual infection rate for cardiovascular implants and orthopedic implants, that is, 7.4 and 4.3% respectively, in USA hospital settings. Unfortunately, data are not available on the concurrent nasal/throat colonization of MRSA as possible patient-implant related factors and DI failure.

Clinical recommendations for avoiding and managing surgical complications associated with implant dentistry have been recently published [150, 151]. However, despite careful planning, infection is one of the early and late implant complications and iatrogenic actions are regarded as accidents during surgical procedures, complications, or failures caused by a deficient praxis of the professional. Infection is the most common explanation for complications such as swelling, suppuration, fistulas, and early/late mucosal dehiscence that may point to implant failure.

Many papers have reported improvements (mainly on the topography and surface features; antimicrobial dental implant functionalization strategies) of DIs and surgery techniques to get better osteointegration and to reduce the infective complications and then to improve long-term success (longevity and function of implants and uploaded prosthesis) [27–30, 32].

Peri-implantitis is a nonspecific, polymicrobial, and heterogeneous diseases of endogenous (caused by commensal oral strains) and iatrogenic nature, with an increased level of pathogenic bacteria from the orange and red complexes and towards a flora with a greater proportion of Gram-negative, motile, anaerobic bacteria [29, 152]. Compared to periodontal disease, the microbial biofilm harbored in peri-implant infective diseases is generally changeable and composed of opportunistic and Gram-negative species. Implant failure can occur at any time during the implant treatment by bacterial infection, but early healing period is quite important due to impaired wound healing.

These microorganisms have been found differently associated to implant infections: *Porphyromonas gingivalis; endodontalis* and *spp.; Tannerella forsythia and socransky; Prevotella nigrescens, oris,* and *intermedia; Fusobacterium* spp. *and nucleatum; Synergistetes* spp. *HO T—360; Pseudoramibacter alactolyticus; Eubacterium* spp.; *Veillonella* spp.; *Enterobacteriaceae; Candida* spp.; *Filifactor alocis; Dialister invisus; Mitsuokella* spp. *HOT 131; Peptococcus* spp. *HO T-168; Clostridiales [F-1] [G-1]* spp. *HO T-093; Catonella morbid; Chloroflexi* spp.; *Tenericutes* spp.; *Aggregatibacter actinomycetemcomitans; Staphylococcus aureus, anaerobius,* and *intermedius; Streptococcus mitis;* spirochete including *Treponema denticola,* with some differences associated to the type of DI and bacterial infiltration in the internal screw threads of implants [29, 153–155]. Moreover, implants with a peri-implant lesion had a higher frequency of superinfecting bacteria, mainly *Klebsiella pneumoniae* and *Burkholderia cepacia,* which are considered environmental and multidrug-resistant bacteria. Significantly higher bacterial counts (*Porphyromonas gingivalis, Tannerella forsythia, Treponema denticola, Prevotella intermedia,* and *Fusobacterium nucleatum*) were found for periodontal pathogenic bacteria within the implant-abutment interface of implants in patients with peri-implantitis compared to those implants surrounded by healthy peri-implant tissues [156]. Using next-generation sequencing methods, recent results indicate that peri-implantitis and periodontitis are both polymicrobial infections with different causative pathogens, and the severity of the peri-implantitis was species-associated, including with *Eubacterium minutum* and an uncultured *Treponema* sp. [157, 158]. Opportunistic microorganisms (enteric rods and *S. aureus*) were found differently in peri-implantitis sites [21, 145].

We underline that some of them (*Enterobacteriaceae, Candida, Staphylococcus, and Streptococcus*) have been indicated as prioritized bacteria in CDC recommendation [18]. Some authors reported that antibiotics do not seem to reduce the incidence of postoperative infections and 2/3 of the infected implants failed before prosthetic loading [21, 146–149]. The majority of bacterial pathogens isolated from peri-implantitis were resistant in vitro to one or more of the tested antibiotics (clindamycin, amoxicillin, doxycycline, or metronidazol) [21].

Nevertheless, microbial investigations seem not contributory to clinician decisions or to be easily applicable nowadays in private practice; the standard procedures (probing, bleeding on probing, probing depth, radiographic assessment, implant mobility) and the visual evaluation of the hyperplastic soft tissues, color changes of the marginal peri-implant tissues, and suppuration are widely used to evaluate the consequences of implant-associated complications [158].

6.2.1 Why does the debridement in dentistry?

Here, we think important to underline some cellular events in relation to implant failures and surgical infections in dentistry. Osseointegration is completed within 3–6 months after implant placement into the dental alveolus, and infection may develop in the early operative period (early infection) or after the process of implant integration (late infection).

At the cellular level, implant-associated infections are the result of two critical phases in the first 6 h post implantation; firstly, the bacterial adhesion to a biomaterial surface by weak and unspecific forces within 1–2 h after implantation, and approximately 2–3 h later, a stronger adhesion with the formation of microcolonies and biofilm, which precedes clinical infection [63]. It is important that *Staphylococcus* species, isolated in dental settings, show high affinity to titanium and good biofilm production [102, 159], which are concurrent detrimental factors for osteogenesis [160, 161]. In addition, during the stationary phase, at least 1% of bacterial cells in biofilms become tolerant to antibiotics [162]. Moreover, the extracellular matrix should provide a stable physical environment for cell to-cell contact, which allows the dissemination of antibiotic resistance by horizontal gene transfer among *S. aureus* [163].

In is well known that smoking is associated with DI failures [159] and that some infective agents (i.e. *Porphyromonas gingivalis*, SA, etc.) showed increased colonization in smokers. Cigarette smoking induces Staphylococcal biofilm formation in an oxidant-dependent manner and enhancement of fibronectin, an important extracellular matrix protein, binding in *S. aureus* [164]. This is relevant for adherence, invasion, and colonization since Staphylococci, in particular *S. aureus*, are the main causes of bone infections [165]. In addition, by molecular mechanisms, *Staphylococci* are able to invade *in vivo* host bone cells (osteoblasts and osteocytes), endothelial cells, and the canaliculi of live cortical bone leading to biofilm formation in osteocyte lacunae [166]. *Staphylococci,* as facultative intracellular pathogens, are shielded from immune response and antibiotics and are expected to induce a highly programmed and regulated cell death of osteogenic cells and then to impair bone formation. *E. faecalis* too is capable of surviving in a vegetative state in healed bone and of reactivation upon DI placement [22].

Then, it is not surprising that a nightmare and a difficult problem are to eradicate implant infections in present dental practice [149]. For the success of the DI surgery, it seems important a careful debridement of the alveolus from infective agents, frequently drug resistants, above all in the case of immediate DI loading after dental extraction and to defer DI placement after a dental extraction [27, 167].

6.3 Focus on orthodontia-associated surgery

Infections complications in orthognathic surgery are lower only to those caused by nerve injury [168]. The incidence of surgical site infections was limited to 1% of patients after bimaxillary orthognathic, osseous genioplasty, and intranasal surgery and under antibiotic treatment [162]. No attention is given to ARIAs in orthodontia and orthognathic surgery. To date, there is no gold standard for the treatment of postoperative infections in orthodontic surgery and the use of prophylactic antibiotics before some orthodontic procedures (orthodontic band placement, separator placement, or screw insertion) in patients with a medical history that reveals the presence of diseases affecting the host defense system (aging, patient on corticosteroids or bisphosphonates or anticoagulants, diabetes mellitus, HIV/AIDS) since they are at high risk of developing oral infection [37, 169]. Endocarditic prophylaxis is indicated only during the initial placement of orthodontic bands (not brackets).

We previously reviewed the problems related to task-specific evidence-based guidelines for cross-infection control when placing different temporary orthodontic anchorage devices [37]. Infection occurred in 17.3% of the installed miniplates and was caused by predominantly anaerobic, mainly Gram-negative bacteria and associated to immune aging [37, 170, 171]. The failure rate of mini-implants is about threefold to fivefold higher than that of dental implants and mini-plates; nevertheless, the mechanism that leads to mobility and then to their clinical failure is still unknown and more tricky to understand [172]. Recently, interest is arising on the use of antibiotics/antiseptics for some potential beneficial effects on tooth stability after orthodontic treatment, but the advantages should be very carefully balanced in accordance with the risk of antibiotic resistance [173].

7. Conclusion

Human infectious diseases will be never-ending [174]. After limitation of dental benefits, there was an increase in the volume and severity of odontogenic infections, surgical cares increased 100%, and the related healthcare cost skyrockets [175]. The reported data show that opportunistic species and/or ARIA infections are nearby and expected to increase in dental setting [21–26, 29, 81, 82, 85, 91–99, 101–105, 109–114, 120–124, 136–141, 145–149, 153–155, 159, 160, 165] due to the overuse of antibiotics in dentistry and the limited awareness on infection prevention guidelines and the lapses and errors during infection prevention [176]. Moreover, it is considered alarming the genetic connection or similarity between MRSAs isolated in dental clinics and on dentures and the EMRSA-15 or EMRSA-16 clone [97, 102, 119]. In addition, Enterobacteriaceae and some resistant strains are present in oral cavity of dental patients, and recently, the transmission in dental practice has been proven [11, 120–124]. The incidence rate of enterococcal endocarditis among the total patient population at the oral surgery practice has been reported to be more than 200 times the expected rate among general population [11].

Then, dental teams have to face occupational and clinical hazards due to ARIA infections in dental facilities. In the absence of or limited new effective antibiotic discovery, the sustainable use of antibiotics is essential but have delayed significant effects [177] based on many collective actions (people information, professional dental-care providers, policy-maker and regulators, industry stakeholders). On the contrary, the prevention of cross infection by adopting guidelines is easily applicable and has had early significant effects on infection prevention and cost-saving [178, 179]. Moreover, it is basic to safeguard dental team reputation, insurance coverings, and reimbursements [8–11, 33–42, 176] and to limit the nightmares to get rid of current dental implant infections [149].

Conflict of interest

L.B. had a service agreement with KerrHawe and is a consultant for Dental Trey Il Blog (http://blog.dentaltrey.it/), neither of which gave any input or financial support to the writing of this article. There are no other conflicts of interest to report.

Abbreviations

AE	adverse event
ARIA	antibiotic-resistant infectious agents
CAGR	compound annual growth rate
CA-MRSA	community-acquired MRSA
CDC	Centers for Disease Control and Prevention
CCSs	clinical contact surfaces
cna	collagen
DD	dental device
DHCP	dental healthcare personnel
DI	dental implant
DOI	delayed-onset infections
DUWL	dental unit water line
eHOMD	expanded human oral microbiome database
EMRSA	epidemic MRSA
EPS	extracellular polysaccharides
FAE	fatal adverse event
fnb	fibronectin
GBR	guided bone regeneration
HA	hospital-acquired

HA-MRSA	hospital-acquired MRSA
HCW	healthcare workers
HPC	heterotrophic plate count
ica	*intercellular adhesion*
HSV	herpes simplex virus
IFU	instruction for use
MAUDE	manufacturer and user facility device experience database
MRSA	methicillin-resistant *Staphylococcus aureus*
PCR	polymerase chain reaction
VRE	vancomycin-resistant *Enterococcus*

Author details

Livia Barenghi[1*], Alberto Barenghi[1] and Alberto Di Blasio[2]

1 Integrated Orthodontic Services S.r.l., Lecco, Italy

2 Department of Medicine and Surgery, Centro di Odontoiatria, Parma University, Parma, Italy

*Address all correspondence to: livia.barenghi@libero.it

IntechOpen

References

[1] Heballi NB, Ramoni R, Kalenderian E, Delattre VF, Stewart DCL, Kent K, et al. The danger of dental devices as reported in the FDA MAUDE database. The Journal of the American Dental Association. 2015;**142**(2):102-110. DOI: 10.1016/J.adaj.2014.11.015

[2] Nalliah RP. Trends in US malpractice payments in dentistry compared to other health professions—Dentistry payments increase, others fall. British Dental Journal. 2017;**222**:36-40. DOI: 10.1038/sj.bdj.2017.34

[3] Hiivala N. Patient safety incidents, their contributing, and mitigating factors in dentistry [thesis]. Universitatis Helsinkiensis; 2016

[4] Ramoni R, Walji M. Creating a dental patient safety initiative. In: Proceedings of the Organization for Safety, Asepsis and Prevention Symposium (OSAP 2015); 28-30 May 2015; Baltimore. Available from: https://www.osap. org. [Accessed: Jun 10, 2015]

[5] Kalenderian E, Obadan-Udoh E, Maramaldi P, Etolue J, Yansane A, Stewart D, et al. Classifying adverse events in the dental office. Journal of Patient Safety. 2017;**00**:00-00. DOI: 10.1097/PTS.0000000000000407

[6] Summary of Infection Prevention Practices in Dental Settings. USA: Centers for Disease Control and Prevention; 2016. Available from: www. cdc.gov/oralhealth/infectioncontrol/pdf/ safe-care2.pdf [Accessed: Jun 12, 2018]

[7] Reuter NG, Westgate PM, Ingram M, Miller CS. Death related to dental treatment: A systematic review. Oral Surgery Oral Medicine Oral Pathology Oral Radiology. 2016;**123**(2):194-204. DOI: 10.1016/j.oooo.2016.10.015

[8] Cleveland JL, Gray SK, Harte JA, Robison VA, Moorman AC, Gooch BF. Transmission of blood-borne pathogens in us dental health care settings. 2016 Update. The Journal of the American Dental Association. 2016;**147**(9):729-738. DOI: 10.1016/j.adaj.2016.03.02

[9] Arduino M, Miller J, Shannon M. Safe water, safe dentistry, safe kids. Organization for Safety, Asepsis and Prevention. Webinar. Available from: https://www.osap.org/page/ LecturesWebinarsConf. [Accessed: May 27, 2017]

[10] Ricci ML, Ricci ML, Fontana S, Pinci F, Fiumana E, Pedna MF, et al. Pneumonia associated with a dental unit water line. The Lancet. 2012;**379**(9816):684. DOI: 10.1016/ S0140-6736(12)60074-9

[11] Ross KM, Mehr JS, Greeley RD, Montoya LA, Kulkarni PTA, Frontin S, et al. Outbreak of bacterial endocarditis associated with an oral surgery practice. The Journal of the American Dental Association. 2018;**149**(3):191-201. DOI: 10.1016/j.adaj.2017.10.002

[12] Perea-Perez B, Labajo-Gonzalez E, Acosta-Gio AE, Yamalik N. Eleven basic procedures/practices for dental patient safety. Journal of Patient Safety. 2015;**00**:00-00. DOI: 10.1097/ PTS.0000000000000234

[13] Davies DS. Dental news. British Dental Journal. 2013;**214**(7):329

[14] Petti S, Polimeni A. Risk of methicillin-resistant *Staphylococcus aureus* transmission in the dental healthcare setting: A narrative review. Infection Control and Hospital Epidemiology. 2011;**32**(11):1109-1115. DOI: 10.1086/662184

[15] Laheij AMGA, Kistler JO, Belibasakis GN, Välimaa H, de Soet JJ. Healthcare-associated viral and bacterial infections in dentistry. Journal

of Oral Microbiology. 2012;**4**(1):17659.
DOI: 10.3402/jom.v4i0.17659

[16] Bell BG, Schellevis F, Stobberingh
E, Goossens H, Pringle M. Systematic
review and meta-analysis of the
effects of antibiotic consumption
on antibiotic resistance. BMC
Infectious Diseases. 2014;**14**:13. DOI:
10.1186/1471-2334-14-13

[17] Merlos A, Vinuesa T, Jane-Salas E,
Lopez-Lopez J, Vinas M. Antimicrobial
prophylaxis in dentistry. Journal of
Global Antimicrobial Resistance.
2014;**2**:232-238. DOI: 10.1016/j.
jgar.2014.05.007 2213-7165

[18] Centers for Disease Control and
Prevention, Office of Infectious
Disease. Antibiotic Resistance Threats
in the United States, 2013. April 2013.
Available from: http://www.cdc.gov/
drugresistance/threat-report-2013
[Accessed: Jul 24, 2018]

[19] Ventola CL. The antibiotic
resistance crisis. Part 1: Causes and
threats. Pharmacy and Therapeutics.
2015;**40**(4):277-283

[20] Ventola CL. The antibiotic
resistance crisis. Part 2: Management
strategies and new agents. Pharmacy
and Therapeutics. 2015;**40**(5):344-352

[21] Rams TE, Degener JE, van
Winkenlhoff AJ. Antibiotic resistance
in human peri-implantitis microbiota.
Clinical Oral Implants Research.
2014;**25**:82-90. DOI: 10.1111/clr.12160

[22] Flanagan D. *Enterococcus faecalis*
and dental implants. Journal of Oral
Implantology. 2017;**153**(1):8-11. DOI:
10.1563/aaid-joi-D-16-00069

[23] Rams TE, Degener JE, van
Winkelhoff AJ. Antibiotic resistance
in human chronic periodontitis
microbiota. Journal of Periodontology.
2014;**85**:160-169. DOI: 10.1902/
jop.2013.130142

[24] Ardila CM, Granada MI, Guzmàn
IC. Antibiotic resistance of subgingival
species in chronic periodontitis patients.
Journal of Periodontal Research.
2010;**45**:557-563

[25] Sun J, Song X, Kristiansen BE,
Kjæreng A, Willems RJL, Eriksen
HM, et al. Occurrence, population
structure, and antimicrobial resistance
of *Enterococci* in marginal and apical
periodontitis. Journal of Clinical
Microbiology. 2009;**47**(7):2218-2225.
DOI: 10.1128/JCM.00388-09

[26] Dahlén G, Blomquist S, Carlén
A. A retrospective study on the
microbiology in patients with oral
complaints and oral mucosal lesions.
Oral Diseases. 2009;**15**:265-272. DOI:
10.1111/j.1601-0825.2009.01520.x

[27] Elias CN, Meirelles L. Improving
osseointegration of dental implants.
Expert Review of Medical Devices.
2010;**7**(2):241-256. DOI: 10.1586/
ERD.09.74

[28] Duraccio D, Mussano F, Faga
MG. Biomaterials for dental implants:
Current and future trends. Journal of
Materials Science. 2015;**50**:4779-4812.
DOI: 10.1007/s10853-015-9056-3

[29] Pokrowiecki R, Mielczarek A,
Zaręba T, Tyski S. Oral microbiome and
peri-implant diseases: Where are we
now? Therapeutics and Clinical Risk
Management. 2017;**13**:1529-1542. DOI:
10.2147/TCRM.S139795

[30] Rasouli R, Barhoum A, Uludag H.
A review of nanostructured surfaces
and materials for dental implants:
Surface coating, patterning and
functionalization for improved
performance. Biomaterials Science.
2018;**6**:1312-1338. DOI: 10.1039/
c8bm00021b

[31] Dental Implants Market Size,
Share & Trends Analysis Report By
Product (Titanium Implants, Zirconium

Implants), By Region (North America, Europe, Asia Pacific, Latin America, MEA), and Segment Forecasts, 2011-2024. [Internet]. Available from: https://www.grandviewresearch.com/industry-analysis/dental-implants-market [Accessed: Apr 15, 2018]

[32] Pjetursson BE, Asgeirsson AG, Zwahlen M, Sailer I. Improvements in implant dentistry over the last decade: Comparison of survival and complication rates in older and newer publications. International Journal of Oral and Maxillofacial Implants. 2014;**29**(8 Suppl):308-324. DOI: 10.11607/jomi.2014suppl.g5.2

[33] Chang W-J, Chang Y-H. Patient satisfaction analysis: Identifying key drivers and enhancing service quality of dental care. Journal of Dental Sciences. 2013;**8**:239-247. DOI: 10.1016/j.jds.2012.10.006

[34] Clayton JL, Miller KJ. Professional and regulatory infection control guidelines: Collaboration to promote patient safety. AORN Journal. 2017;**106**:201-210. DOI: 10.1016/j.aorn.2017.07.005

[35] Collins FM. The significance of the US Food and Drug Administration for dental professionals and safe patient care. The Journal of the American Dental Association. 2017;**148**(11):858-861. DOI: 10.1016/j.adaj.2017.08.026

[36] Oosthuysen J, Potgieter E, Fossey A. Compliance with infection prevention and control in oral health-care facilities: A global perspective. International Dental Journal. 2014;**64**(6):297-311. DOI: 10.1111/idj.12134

[37] Barenghi L, Barenghi A, Di Blasio A. Implementation of recent infection prevention procedures published by centers for disease control and prevention: Difficulties and problems in orthodontic offices. Iranian Journal of Orthodontics. 2018;**13**(1):e10201. DOI: 10.5812/ijo.10201

[38] Barenghi L. Clean, disinfect and cover: Top activities for clinical contact surfaces in dentistry [Internet]. 2015. Available from: www.kerrdental.com/resource-center/clean-disinfect-and-cover-%E2%80%93top-activities-clinical-contactsurfaces-dentistry-dr [Accessed: Jun 12, 2018]

[39] Barenghi L. The Daily Fight to Limit Cross-infection in a Dental Office [Internet]. 2017. Webinar. Available from: http://blog.kavo.com/en/webinar-daily-fight-limit-cross-infection-dental-office [Accessed: Jun 12, 2018]

[40] Jakubovics N, Greenwood M, Meechan JG. General medicine and surgery for dental practitioners: Part 4. Infections and infection control. British Dental Journal. 2014;**217**(2):73-77. DOI: 10.1038/sj.bdj.2014.593

[41] Monarca S, Grottolo M, Renzi D, Paganelli C, Sapelli P, Zerbini I, et al. Evaluation of environmental bacterial contamination and procedures to control cross infection in a sample of Italian dental surgeries. Occupational and Environmental Medicine. 2000;**57**:721-726. DOI: 10.1136/oem.57.11.721

[42] Schaefer MK, Michael J, Marilyn Dahl M, et al. Infection control assessment of ambulatory surgical centers. Journal of the American Medical Association. 2010;**303**(22):2273-2279. DOI: 10.1001/jama.2010.744

[43] Ehrlich T, Dietz B. Chapter 30. In: Modern Dental Assisting. 5th ed. USA: W.B. Sounders Company; 1995. ISBN: 0-7216-5053-8

[44] Miller CH, Palenik CJ. Chapters 14, 17. In: Infection Control and Management of Hazardous Materials for the Dental Team. 4th ed. Evolve. USA: Mosby Elsevier; 2010. ISBN: 978-0-323-05631-1

[45] Pankhurst CL, Coulter WA. Chapters 2, 4-9. In: Basic Guide to

Infection Prevention and Control in Dentistry. 2nd ed. UK: Wiley Blackwell; 2017. ISBN: 9781119164982

[46] Rutala WA, Weber DJ. The Healthcare Infection Control Practices Advisory Committee (HICPAC). Guidelines for Infection Control in Dental Health-Care Settings 2003–MMVR 2003521-61. Available from: www.cdc. gov/mnwr/preview/mmwrhtlm/rr5217al. htm [Accessed: Jun 12, 2018]

[47] Rutala WA, Weber DJ, The Healthcare Infection Control Practices Advisory Committee (HICPAC). Guideline for Disinfection and Sterilization in Healthcare Facilities. 2008. Available from: www.cdc.gov/ infectioncontrol/quidelines/disinfection [Accessed: Feb 15, 2017]

[48] Expanded Human Oral Microbiome Database (eHOMD). Available from: www.homd.org/index.php [Accessed: May 18, 2018]

[49] Siqueira JF, Fouad AF, Rocas IN. Pyrosequencing as a tool for better understanding of human microbiomes. Journal of Oral Microbiology. 2012;**4**:10743. DOI: 10.3402/jom. v4i0.10743

[50] Tsunemine H, Yoshioka Y, Nagao M, Tomaru Y, Saitoh T, Adachi S, et al. Multiplex polymerase chain reaction assay for early diagnosis of viral infection. In: Samadikuchaksaraei A, editor. Polymerase Chain Reaction for Biomedical Applications. UK: InTech; 2016. pp. 69-82. DOI: 10.5772/65771

[51] Rozman U, Turk SŠ. PCR technique for the microbial analysis of inanimate hospital environment. In: Samadikuchaksaraei A, editor. Polymerase Chain Reaction for Biomedical Applications. UK: InTech; 2016. pp. 119-134. DOI: 10.5772/65742

[52] Valeriani F, Protano C, Gianfranceschi G, Cozza P, Campanella

V, Liguori G, et al. Infection control in healthcare settings: Perspectives for mfDNA analysis in monitoring sanitation procedures. BMC Infectious Diseases. 2016;**16**:394. DOI: 10.1186/ s12879-016-1714-9

[53] Lamas A, Franco CM, Regal P, Miranda JM, Vázquez B, Cepeda A. High-throughput platforms in real-time PCR and applications. In: Samadikuchaksaraei A, editor. Polymerase Chain Reaction for Biomedical Applications. UK: InTech; 2016. pp. 15-38. DOI: 10.5772/65760

[54] Kouidhi B, Zmantar T, Mahdouani K, Hentati H, Bakhrouf A. Antibiotic resistance and adhesion properties of oral *Enterococci* associated to dental caries. BMC Microbiology. 2011;**11**:155. DOI: 10.1186/1471-2180-11-155

[55] Tsang STJ, McHugh MP, Guerendiain D, Gwynne PJ, Boyd J, Simpson AHRW, et al. Underestimation of *Staphylococcus aureus* (MRSA and MSSA) carriage associated with standard culturing techniques. Bone & Joint Research. 2018;7:79-84. DOI: 10.1302/2046-3758.71.BJR2017-0175.R1

[56] Charalampakis G, Leonhardt A, Rabe P, Dahlen G. Clinical and microbiological characteristics of peri-implantitis cases: A retrospective multicentre study. Clinical Oral Implants Research. 2012;**23**:1045-1054. DOI: 10.1111/j.1600-0501.2011.02258.x

[57] Korkut E, Uncu AT, Sener Y. Biofilm formation by *Staphylococcus aureus* isolates from a dental clinic in Konya, Turkey. Journal of Infection and Public Health. 2017;**10**:809-813. DOI: 10.1016/j. jiph.2017.01.004

[58] Siqueira JF, Rocas IN. Polymerase chain reaction-based analysis of microorganisms associated with failed endodontic treatment. Oral Surgery Oral Medicine Oral Pathology Oral

Radiology. 2004;**97**:85-94. DOI: 10.1016/S1079210403003536

[59] Pankhurst C, Rautemaa-Richardson R, Seoudi N, Smith A, Wilson M. Antibiotics and consultant oral microbiologist posts. British Dental Journal. 2016;**220**(1):2-3. DOI: 10.1038/sj.bdj.2016.5

[60] Emecen-Huja P, Hasan I, Miller CS. Biologic markers of failing implants. Dental Clinics. 2015;**59**(1):179-194. DOI: 10.1016/j.cden.2014.08.007

[61] Hoyos-Nogués M, Brosel-Oliu S, Abramova N, Muñoz F-X, Bratov A, Mas-Moruno C, et al. Impedimetric antimicrobial peptide-based sensor for the early detection of periodontopathogenic bacteria. Biosensors and Bioelectronics. 2016;**15**(86):377-385. DOI: 10.1016/j.bios.2016.06.066

[62] Salako NO, Rotimib VO, Adibb SM, Al-Mutawac S. Pattern of antibiotic prescription in the management of oral diseases among dentists in Kuwait. Journal of Dentistry. 2004;**32**:503-509. DOI: 10.1016/j.jdent.2004.04.001

[63] Monteiro Lisboa S, Parreiras M, de Castilho LS, de Souza e Silva ME, Nogueira Guimarães AM. Prescribing errors in antibiotic prophylaxis by dentists in a large Brazilian city. American Journal of Infection Control. 2015;**43**:767-768. DOI: 10.1016/j.ajic.2015.03.028

[64] Marra F, George D, Chong M, Sutherland S, Patrick DM. Antibiotic prescribing by dentists has increased. Why? The Journal of the American Dental Association. 2016;**147**(5):320-327. DOI: 10.1016/j.adaj.2015.12.014

[65] Haliti N, Krasniqi S, Begzati A, Gllareva B, Krasniqi L, Shabani N, et al. Antibiotic prescription patterns in primary dental health care in Kosovo. Family Medicine & Primary Care Review. 2017;**19**, 2:128-133. DOI: 10.5114/fmpcr.2017.67866

[66] Loffler C, Bohmer F. The effect of interventions aiming to optimize the prescription of antibiotics in dental care—A systematic review. PLoS One. 2017;**12**(11):e0188061. DOI: 10.1371/journal.pone.0188061

[67] Buttar R, Aleksejuniene J, Shen Y, Coil J. Antibiotic and opioid analgesic prescribing patterns of dentists in vancouver and endodontic specialists in British Columbia. Journal of the Canadian Dental Association. 2017;**83**:h8. PMID: 29513210

[68] Koyuncuoglu CZ, Aydin M, Kirmizi NI, Aydin V, Aksoy M, Isli F, et al. Rational use of medicine in dentistry: Do dentists prescribe antibiotics in appropriate indications? European Journal of Clinical Pharmacology. 2017;**73**:1027-1032. DOI: 10.1007/s00228-017-2258-7

[69] Prasad S, Rajesvari R. Antibiotic prescribing practice among general dental practitioners. Journal of Oral Medicine, Oral Surgery, Oral Pathology and Oral Radiology. 2017;**3**(1):14-16. DOI: 10.18231/2395-6194.2017.0004

[70] Oteri G, Panzarella V, Marciano A, Di Fede O, Maniscalco L, Peditto M, et al. Appropriateness in dentistry: A survey discovers improper procedures in oral medicine and surgery. International Journal of Dentistry. 2018;**00**:10 Article ID 3245324. DOI: 10.1155/2018/3245324

[71] Khalil D, Lund B, Hultin M. Antibiotics in implant dentistry. In: Mazen Ahmad M, Almasri JA, editors. Dental Implantology and Biomaterial. UK: InTech; 2016. pp. 19-38. DOI: 10.5772/62681

[72] Swedres-Svarm. Consumption of antibiotics and occurrence of resistance in Sweden. Solna/Uppsala. 2016. ISSN: 1650-6332. Available from: www.

folkhalsomyndigheten.se/contentassets/
d118ac95c12d4c11b3e61d34ee6d2332/
swedres-svarm-2016-16124.pdf
[Accessed: Jun 16, 2018]

[73] Holmstrup P, Klausen B. The
growing problem of antimicrobial
resistance. Oral Diseases. 2018;**24**:291-
295. DOI: 10.1111/odi.12610

[74] Martins JR, Chagas OL, Velasques
BD, Niemczewski Bobrowski A, Britto
Correa M, Torriani MA. The use of
antibiotics in odontogenic infections:
What is the best choice? A systematic
review. Journal of Oral and Maxillofacial
Surgery. 2017;**75**:2606.e1-2606.e11. DOI:
10.1016/j.joms.2017.08.017

[75] Segura-Egea JJ, Gould K, Hakan Sen
B, Jonasson P, Cotti E, Mazzoni A, et al.
European Society of Endodontology
position statement: The use of
antibiotics in endodontics. International
Endodontic Journal. 2018;**51**:20-25. DOI:
10.1111/iej.12781

[76] Ramos E, Santamaría J, Santamaría
G, Barbier L, Arteagoitia I. Do systemic
antibiotics prevent dry socket and
infection after third molar extraction?
A systematic review and meta-
analysis. Oral Surgery Oral Medicine
Oral Pathology Oral Radiology.
2016;**122**:403-425. DOI: 10.1016/j.
oooo.2016.04.016

[77] Bailey E, Tickle M, Campbell S,
O'Malley L. Systematic review of patient
safety interventions in dentistry. BMC
Oral Health. 2015;**15**:152. DOI: 10.1186/
s12903-015-0136-1

[78] Cloitre A, Duval X, Hoen B,
Alla F, MD LP. A nationwide survey
of French dentists' knowledge and
implementation of current guidelines
for antibiotic prophylaxis of infective
endocarditis in patients with
predisposing cardiac conditions. Oral
Surgery Oral Medicine Oral Pathology
Oral Radiology. 2018;**125**:295-303. DOI:
10.1016/j.oooo.2017.10.002

[79] Dayer M, Thornhill M. Is antibiotic
prophylaxis to prevent infective
endocarditis worthwhile? Journal
of Infection and Chemotherapy.
2018;**24**. DOI: 18e24. DOI: 10.1016/j.
jiac.2017.10.006 1341-321X

[80] ADA Expert Panel. American
Dental Association guidance for
utilizing appropriate use criteria in the
management of the care of patients with
orthopedic implants undergoing dental
procedures. 2017;**148**(2):57-59. DOI:
10.1016/j.adaj.2016.12.002

[81] Hetrick EM, Schoenfisch
MH. Reducing implant-related
infections: Active release strategies.
Chemical Society Reviews. 2006;**35**:780-
789. DOI: 10.1039/b515219b

[82] Miranda-Rius J, Lahor-Soler
E, Brunet-Llobet L, de Dios D, Gil
FX. Treatments to optimize dental
implant surface topography and
enhance cell bioactivity. In: Almasri
MA, editor. Dental Implantology and
Biomaterial. UK: InTech; 2016. pp. 110-
127. DOI: 10.5772/62682

[83] Toledo-Arana A, Valle J, Solano C,
Arrizubieta M, Cucarella C, Lamata
M, et al. The enterococcal surface
protein, Esp, is involved in *Enterococcus
faecalis* biofilm formation. Applied
and Environmental Microbiology.
2001;**67**(10):4538-4545. DOI: 10.1128/
AEM.67.10.4538-4545.2001

[84] Khalil D. The use of antibiotic
prophylaxis in implant dentistry. A
microbiological and clinical perspective
[thesis]. Stockholm, Sweden: Karolinska
Institutet; 2017

[85] Duran-Pinedo AE, Frias-Lopez
J. Beyond microbial community
composition: Functional activities of
the oral microbiome in human health
and disease. Microbes and Infection.
2015;**17**(7):505-516. DOI: 10.1016/j.
micinf.2015.03.014

[86] van der Waaij D, Nord CE. Development and persistence of multi-resistance to antibiotics in bacteria: An analysis and a new approach to this urgent problem. International Journal of Antimicrobial Agents. 2000;**16**(3):191-197

[87] Gordon RJ, Lowy FD. Pathogenesis of methicillin-resistant *Staphylococcus aureus* infection. Clinical Infectious Diseases. 2008;**46**(Suppl 5):S350-S359. DOI: 10.1086/533591

[88] Mertz D, Frei R, Jaussi B, Tietz A, Stebler C, Fluckiger U, et al. Throat swabs are necessary to reliably detect carriers of *Staphylococcus aureus*. Clinical Infectious Diseses. 2007;**45**(4): 475-477. DOI: 10.1086/520016

[89] Abreu AC, Tavares RR, Borges A, Mergulhão F, Simões M. Current and emergent strategies for disinfection of hospital environments. Journal of Antimicrobial Chemotherapy. 2013;**68**:2718-2732. DOI: 10.1093/jac/dkt281

[90] Costalonga M, Herzberg MC. The oral microbiome and the immunobiology of periodontal disease and caries. Immunology Letters. 2014;**162**(200):22-38. DOI: 10.1016/j.imlet.2014.08.017

[91] Roberts MC, Soge OO, Horst JA, Ly KA, Milgrom P. Methicillin-resistant *Staphylococcus aureus* from dental school clinic surfaces and students. American Journal of Infection Control. 2011;**39**:628-632. DOI: 10.1016/j.ajic.2010.11.007

[92] Martınez-Ruız FJ, Carrillo-Espındola TY, Bustos-Martınez J, Hamdan-Partida A, Sanchez-Perez L, Acosta-Gıo AE. Higher prevalence of methicillin-resistant *Staphylococcus aureus* among dental students. Journal of Hospital Infection. 2014;**86**(3): 216-218. DOI: 10.1016/j.jhin.2013.12.00

[93] Petti S, Kakisina N, Volgenant CMC, Messano GA, Barbato E, Passariello C, et al. Low methicillin-resistant *Staphylococcus aureus* carriage rate among Italian dental students. American Journal of Infection Control. 2015;**43**:e89-e91. DOI: org/10.1016/j.ajic.2015.08.00

[94] Baek YS, Baek S-H, Yoo Y-J. Higher nasal carriage rate of methicillin-resistant *Staphylococcus aureus* among dental students who have clinical experience. Journal of the American Dental Association. 2016;**147**(5):348-353. DOI: 10.1016/j.adaj.2015.12.004

[95] Hema N, Raj NS, Chaithanya ED, Chincholi R, Iswariya M, Hema KN. Prevalence of nasal carriers of methicillin-resistant *Staphylococcus aureus* among dental students: An in vivo study. Journal of Oral and Maxillofacial Pathology. 2017;**21**(3):356-359. DOI: 10.4103/jomfp.JOMFP_212_17

[96] Zimmerli M, Widmer AF, Dangel M, Filippi A, Frei R, Meyer J. Methicillin-resistant *Staphylococcus aureus* (MRSA) among dental patients: A problem for infection control in dentistry? Clinical Oral Investigations. 2009;**13**:369-373. DOI: 10.1007/s00784-008-0244-2

[97] McCormack MG, Smith AJ, Akram AN, Jackson M, Robertson D, Edwards MB. *Staphylococcus aureus* and the oral cavity: An overlooked source of carriage and infection? American Journal of Infection Control. 2015;**43**(1):35-37. DOI: 10.1016/j.ajic.2014.09.015

[98] Kabanova A. Bacterial spectrum of orofacial infections and their antibiotic resistance in Belarus. Medical Research Journal. 2017;**2**(4):152-156. DOI: 10.5603/MRJ.2017.0021

[99] Dulon M, Peters C, Schablon A, Nienhaus A. MRSA carriage among healthcare workers in non-outbreak settings in Europe and the United

States: A systematic review. BMC
Infectious Diseases. 2014;**14**:363. DOI:
10.1186/1471-2334-14-363

[100] Esposito S, Terranova L, Ruggiero
L, Ascolese B, Montinaro V, Peves Rios
W, et al. Streptococcus pneumoniae
and Staphylococcus aureus carriage
in healthy school-age children and
adolescents. Journal of Medical
Microbiology. 2015;**64**:427-431. DOI:
10.1099/jmm.0.000029

[101] Koukos G, Sakellari D, Arsenakis
M, Tsalikis L, Slini T, Konstantinidis
A. Prevalence of Staphylococcus
aureus and methicillin resistant
Staphylococcus aureus (MRSA) in the
oral cavity. Archives of Oral Biology.
2015;**60**:1410-1415. DOI: 10.1016/j.
archoralbio.2015.06.009

[102] Kharialla AS, Wasfi R, Ashour
HM. Carriage frequency, phenotypic
and genomic characteristics of
methicillin-resistant Staphylococcus
aureus isolated from dental health care
personnel, patients and environment.
Scientific Reports. 2017;**7**:7390. DOI:
10.1038/s41598-017-07713-8

[103] Yoo Y-J, Kwak E-J, Jeong KM, Baek
S-H, Baek YS. Knowledge, attitudes and
practices regarding methicillinresistant
Staphylococcus aureus (MRSA) infection
control and nasal MRSA carriage rate
among dental health-care professionals.
International Dental Journal. 2018;**00**
:1-8. DOI: 10.1111/idj.12388

[104] Didilescu AC, Skaug N, Marica C,
Didilescu C. Respiratory pathogens in
dental plaque of hospitalized patients
with chronic lung diseases. Clinical Oral
Investigations. 2005;**9**:141-147

[105] Smith AJ, Robertson D, Tang MK,
Jackson MS, MacKenzie D, Bagg J.
Staphylococcus aureus in the oral cavity:
A three year retrospective analysis of
clinical laboratory data. British Dental
Journal. 2003;**195**(12):701-703. DOI:
10.1038/sj.bdj.4810832

[106] Merghni A, Nejma MB, Hentati
H, Mahjoub A, Mastouri M. Adhesive
properties and extracellular enzymatic
activity of Staphylococcus aureus
strains isolated from oral cavity.
Microbial Pathogenesis. 2014;**73**:7-12.
DOI: 10.1016/j.micpath.2014.05.002
0882-4010

[107] Merghni A, Nejma MB, Helali
I, Hentati H, Bongiovanni A, Lafont
F, et al. Assessment of adhesion,
invasion and cytotoxicity potential
of oral Staphylococcus aureus strains.
Microbial Pathogenesis. 2015;**86**:1-9.
DOI: 10.1016/j.micpath.2015.05.010
0882-4010

[108] Suzuki J, Yoshimura G, Kadomoto
N, Kuramoto M, Kozai K. Long-term
periodical isolation of Staphylococcus
aureus and methicillin-resistant
Staphylococcus aureus (MRSA)
from Japanese children's oral
cavities. Pediatric Dental Journal.
2007;**17**(2):127-130. DOI: 10.11411/
pdj.17.127

[109] Merghni A, Nejma MB, Dallel
I, Tobji S, Amor AB, Janel S, et al.
High potential of adhesion to biotic
and abiotic surfaces by opportunistic
Staphylococcus aureus strains
isolated from orthodontic appliances.
Microbial Pathogenesis. 2016;**91**:61-67.
DOI: 10.1016/j.micpath.2015.11.009
0882-4010

[110] Peterson SN, Meissner T, Su AI,
Snesrud E, Ong AC, Schork NJ, et al.
Functional expression of dental plaque
microbiota. Frontiers in Cellular and
Infection Microbiology. 2014;**4**(108):
1-13. DOI: 10.3389/fcimb.2014.00108

[111] Abe S, Ishihara K, Okuda
K. Prevalence of potential respiratory
pathogens in the mouths of elderly
patients and effects of professional oral
care. Archives of Gerontology
and Geriatrics. 2001;**32**:45-55. DOI:
10.1016/S0167-4943(00)00091-1

[112] El-Solh AA, Pietrantoni C, Bhat A, Okada M, Zambon J, Aquilina A, et al. Colonization of dental plaques: A reservoir of respiratory pathogens for hospital-acquired pneumonia in institutionalized elders. Chest Journal. 2004;**126**(5):1575-1582. DOI: 10.1016/S0012-3692(15)31374-X

[113] Vellappally S, Divakar DD, Al Kheraif AA, Ramakrishnaiah R, Alqahtani A, Dalati MHN, et al. Occurrence of vancomycin-resistant Staphylococcus aureus in the oral cavity of patients with dental caries. Acta Microbiologica et Immunologica Hungarica. 2017;**00**:1-9. DOI: 10.1556/030.64.2017.033

[114] Veloo AC, Seme K, Raangs E, Rurenga P, Singadji Z, Wekema-Mulder G, et al. Antibiotic susceptibility profiles of oral pathogens. International Journal of Antimicrobial Agents. 2012;**40**:450-454. DOI: 10.1016/j.ijantimicag.2012.07.004

[115] Sai N, Laurent C, Strale H, Denis O, Byl B. Efficacy of the decolonization of methicillinresistant *Staphylococcus aureus* carriers in clinical practice. Antimicrobial Resistance and Infection Control. 2015;**4**:56. DOI: 10.1186/s13756-015-0096-x

[116] Otter JA, French GL. Molecular epidemiology of community-associated meticillin-resistant Staphylococcus aureus in Europe. The Lancet Infectious Diseases. 2010;**10**(4):227-239. DOI: 10.1016/S1473-3099(10)70053-0

[117] National and State Healthcare Associated Infections. CDC report is based on 2014 data. 2016. Available from: www.cdc.gov/HAI/pdfs/progress-report/hai-progress-report.pdf [Accessed: Jun 16, 2018]

[118] Figueiredo AM. What is behind the epidemiological difference between community-acquired and health-care associated methicillin-resistant

Staphylococcus aureus. Virulence. 2017;**8**(6):640-642. DOI: 10.1080/21505594.2017.1335847

[119] Lewis N, Parmar N, Hussain Z, Baker G, Green I, Howlett J, et al. Colonisation of dentures by *Stap*hylococcus aureus and MRSA in out-patient and in-patient populations. European Journal of Clinical Microbiology & Infectious Diseases. 2015;**34**:1823-1826. DOI: 10.1007/s10096-015-2418-6

[120] Anderson C, Jonas D, Huber I, Karygianni L, Wölber J, Hellwig E, et al. Enterococcus faecalis from food, clinical specimens, and oral sites: Prevalence of virulence factors in association with biofilm formation. Frontiers in Microbiology. 2016;**6**:1534. DOI: 10.3389/fmicb.2015.01534

[121] Komiyama EY, Lepesqueur LSS, Yassuda CG, Samaranayake LP, Parahitiyawa NB, Balducci I, et al. Enterococcus species in the oral cavity: Prevalence, virulence factors and antimicrobial susceptibility. PLoS One. 2016;**11**(9):e0163001. DOI: 10.1371/journal.pone.0163001

[122] Rams TE, Feik D, Mortensen JE, Degener JE, van Winkelhoff AJ. Antibiotic Susceptibility of Periodontal Enterococcus faecalis. Journal of Periodontology. 2013;**84**(7):1026-1033. DOI: 10.1902/jop.2012.120050

[123] O'Driscoll T, Crank CW. Vancomycin-resistant enterococcal infections: Epidemiology, clinical manifestations, and optimal management. Infection and Drug Resistance. 2015;**8**:217-230. DOI: 10.2147/IDR.S54125

[124] Magiorakos AP, Burns K, Baño JR, M Borg M, Daikos G, Dumpis U, et al. Infection prevention and control measures and tools for the prevention of entry of carbapenem-resistant

Enterobacteriaceae into healthcare settings: Guidance from the European Centre for Disease Prevention and Control. Antimicrobial Resistance and Infection Control. 2017;6:113. DOI: 10.1186/s13756-017-0259-z

[125] Tyson GH, Sabo JL, Rice-Trujillo C, Hernandez J, McDermott PF. Whole-genome sequencing based characterization of antimicrobial resistance in Enterococcus. Pathogens and Disease. 2018;76:fty018. DOI: 10.1093/femspd/fty018

[126] Abu-Ta'a M, Quirynen M, Teughels W, van Steenberghe D. Asepsis during periodontal surgery involving oral implants and the usefulness of peri-operative antibiotics: A prospective, randomized, controlled clinical trial. Journal of Clinical Periodontology. 2008;35:58-63. DOI: 10.1111/j.1600-051X.2007.01162.x

[127] Dancer SJ. Controlling hospital-acquired infection: Focus on the role of the environment and new technologies for decontamination. Clinical Microbiology Reviews. 2014;27(4):665-690. DOI: 10.1128/CMR.00020-14

[128] Petti S, Polimeni A, Dancer SJ. Effect of disposable barriers, disinfection, and cleaning on controlling methicillin-resistant Staphylococcus aureus environmental contamination. American Journal of Infection Control. 2013;41(9):836-840. DOI: 10.1016/j.ajic.2012.09.0

[129] Cheng VC-CC, Wong SC-Y, Sridhar S, Chan JF-W, Lai-Ming M, Lau SK-P, et al. Management of an incident of failed sterilization of surgical instruments in a dental clinic in Hong Kong. Journal of the Formosan Medical Association. 2013;112:666-675. DOI: 10.1016/j.jfma.2013.07.020

[130] Neves JK, de Araujo Martins MG, Germinio JES, de Andrade MC, de Oliveira SR. Effectiveness of disinfection of anesthetics tubes in oral surgery-an in vitro study. Journal of Pharmacy and Pharmacology. 2017;7:424-429. DOI: 10.17265/2328-2150/2017.01.005

[131] Hogg NJV, Morrison AD. Resterilization of instruments used in a hospital-based oral and maxillofacial surgery clinic. Journal of Canadian Dental Association. 2005;71:179-182. ISSN: 1488-2159. Available from: www.cda-adc.ca/jcda/vol-71/issue-3/179.html [Accessed: Jul 29, 2017]

[132] Wu G, Yu X. Influence of usage history, instrument complexity, and different cleaning procedures on the cleanliness of blood-contaminated dental surgical instruments. Infection Control and Hospital Epidemiology. 2009;30(7):702-704. DOI: 10.1086/598241

[133] Takamoto M, Takechi M, Ohta K, Ninomiya Y, Ono S, Shigeishi H, et al. Risk of bacterial contamination of bone harvesting devices used for autogenous bone graft in implant surgery. Head & Face Medicine. 2013;9(3):1-5. DOI: 10.1186/1746-160X-9-3

[134] Vassey M, Budge C, Poolman T, Jones P, Perrett D, Nayuni N, et al. A quantitative assessment of residual protein levels on dental instruments reprocessed by manual, ultrasonic and automated cleaning methods. British Dental Journal. 2011;210(9):E14. DOI: 10.1038/sj.bdj.2011.144

[135] Gaetti-Jardim E, Landucci LF, de Oliveira KL, Costa I, Ranieri RV, Okamoto AC, et al. Microbiota associated with infections of the jaws. International Journal of Dentistry. 2012;00:8. Article ID: 369751. DOI: 10.1155/2012/369751

[136] Rega AJ, Aziz SR, Ziccardi VB. Microbiology and antibiotic sensitivities of head and neck space infections of odontogenic origin. Journal of Oral and

Maxillofacial Surgery. 2006;**64**:1377-1380. DOI: 10.1016/j.joms.2006.05.023

[137] Sánchez R, Mirada E, Arias J, Paño JR, Burgueño M. Severe odontogenic infections: Epidemiological, microbiological and therapeutic factors. Medicina Oral Patologia Oral y Cirugia Bucal. 2011;**16**(5):e670-e676. DOI: 10.4317/medoral.16995

[138] Zawadzki BJ, Perkowski K, Padzik M, Mierzwi Nska-Nastalska E, Szaflik JP, Conn DB, et al. Examination of oral microbiota diversity in adults and older adults as an approach to prevent spread of risk factors for human infections. BioMed Research International. 2017;**00**:7. Article ID: 8106491. DOI: 10.1155/2017/8106491

[139] Seppänen L, Lauhio A, Lindqvist C, Suuronen R, Rautemaa R. Analysis of systemic and local odontogenic infection complications requiring hospital care. Journal of Infection. 2008;**57**(2):116-122. DOI: 10.1016/j.jinf.2008.06.002

[140] Opitz D, Camerer C, Camerer D-M, Raguse J-D, Menneking H, Hoffmeister B, et al. Incidence and management of severe odontogenic infections—A retrospective analysis from 2004 to 2011. Journal of Cranio-Maxillofacial Surgery. 2015;**43**(2):285-289. DOI: 10.1016/j.jcms.2014.12.002

[141] Ylijoki S, Suuronen R, Jousimies-Somer H, Meurman JH, Lindqvist C. Differences between patients with or without the need for intensive care due to severe odontogenic infections. Journal of Oral and Maxillofacial Surgery. 2001;**59**(8):867-872. DOI: 10.1053/joms.2001.25017

[142] Navarro BG, Salas EJ, Devesa AE, López JL. Bacteremia associated with oral surgery: A review. Journal of Evidence Based Dental Practice. 2017;**17**(3):190-204. DOI: 10.1016/j.jebdp.2016.12.001

[143] Brunello G, De Biagi M, Crepaldi G, Izaura Rodrigues F, Sivolella S. An observational cohort study on delayed-onset infections after mandibular third-molar extractions. International Journal of Dentistry. 2017;**00**:5. Article ID: 1435348. DOI: 10.1155/2017/1435348

[144] Telles DR, Karki N, Marshall MW. Oral fungal infections diagnosis and management. Dental Clinics of North America. 2017;**61**(2):319-349. DOI: 10.1016/j.cden.2016.12.004

[145] Lafaurie GI, Sabogal MA, Castillo DM, Rincón MV, Gómez LA, Lesmes YA, et al. Microbiome and microbial biolm proles of peri-implantitis: A systematic review. Journal of Periodontology. 2017;**88**(10):1066-1089. DOI: 10.1902/jop.2017.170123

[146] Camps-Font O, Figueiredo R, Valmaseda-Castellón E, Gay-Escoda C. Postoperative infections after dental implant placement: Prevalence, clinical features, and treatment. Implant Dentistry. 2015;**24**(6):713-719. DOI: 10.1097/ID.0000000000000325

[147] Esposito M, Grusovin MG, Worthington HV. Interventions for replacing missing teeth: Antibiotics at dental implant placement to prevent complications. The Cochrane Database of Systematic Reviews. 2013;**31**(7):CD004152. DOI: 10.1002/14651858.CD004152.pub4

[148] Ata-Ali J, Ata-Ali F, Ata-Ali F. Do antibiotics decrease implant failure and postoperative infections? A systematic review and meta-analysis. International Journal of Oral and Maxillofacial Surgery. 2014;**43**(1):68-74. DOI: 10.1016/j.ijom.2013.05.019

[149] Sánchez FR, Andrés CR, Arteagoitia I. Which antibiotic regimen prevents implant failure or infection after dental implant surgery? A systematic review and meta-analysis. Journal of Cranio-Maxillofacial Surgery. 2018;**46**(4):722-736. DOI: 10.1016/j.jcms.2018.02.004

[150] Garcés SMA, Escoda-Francolí J, Gay-Escoda C. Implant complications. In: Turkyilmaz I, editor. Implant Dentistry—The Most Promising Discipline of Dentistry. UK: InTech; 2011. pp. 369-396. DOI: 10.5772/19706

[151] Ucer C, Wright S, Scher E, West N, Retzepi M, Simpson S, et al. ADI Guidelines on Peri-implant Monitoring and Maintenance. 2013. Available from: www.adi.org.uk/resources/guidelines_and_papers/peri-implant/ [Accessed: Jul 24, 2018]

[152] Nandakumar V, Chittaranjan S, Kurian VM, Doble M. Characteristics of bacterial biofilm associated with implant material in clinical practice. Polymer Journal. 2013;45:137-152. DOI: 10.1038/pj.2012.130

[153] Pye AD, Lockhart DEA, Dawson MP, Murray CA, Smith AJ. A review of dental implants and infection. Journal of Hospital Infection. 2009;72:104e110. DOI: 10.1016/j.jhin.2009.02.010

[154] Do Nascimento C, de Albuquerque RF. Bacterial leakage along the implant-abutment interface. In: Implant Dentistry—The Most Promising Discipline of Dentistry. UK: InTech; 2011. DOI: 10.5772/20109

[155] Charalampakis G, Rabe P, Leonhardt A, Dahlen G. A follow-up study of periimplantitis cases after treatment. Journal of Clinical Periodontology. 2011;00:1-8. DOI: 10.1111/j.1600-051X.2011.01759.x

[156] Tallarico M, Canullo L, Caneva M, Özcan M. Microbial colonization at the implant-abutment interface and its possible influence on periimplantitis: A systematic review and meta-analysis. Journal of Prosthodontics. 2017;61(3):233-241. DOI: 10.1016/j.jpor.2017.03.001

[157] Zheng H, Xu L, Wang Z, Li L, Zhang J, Zhang Q, et al. Subgingival microbiome in patients with healthy and ailing dental implants. Scientific Reports. 2015;5(10948):1-11. DOI: 10.1038/srep10948

[158] Maruyama N, Maruyama F, Takeuchi Y, Aikawa C, Izumi Y, Nakagawa I. Intraindividual variation in core microbiota in peri-implantitis and periodontitis. Scientific Reports. 2014;4(6602):1-10. DOI: 10.1038/srep06602

[159] Smeets R, Henningsen A, Jung O, Heiland M, Hammacher C, Stein JM. Definitiom, etiology, prevention and treatment of peri-implantitis-a review. Head & Face Medicine. 2014;10:34. DOI: 10.1186/1746-160X-10-34

[160] Flemming HC, Wingender J, Szewzyk U, Steinberg P, Rice SA, Kjelleberg S. Biofilms: An emergent form of bacterial life. Nature Reviews Microbiology. 2016;14:563-575. DOI: 10.1038/nrmicro.2016.94

[161] Maisonneuve E, Gerdes K. Molecular mechanisms underlying bacterial persisters. Cell. 2014;157(3):539-548. DOI: 10.1016/j.cell.2014.02.050

[162] Posnick JC, Choi E, Chavda A. Surgical site infections following bimaxillary orthognathic, osseous genioplasty, and intranasal surgery: A retrospective Cohort Study. Journal of Oral and Maxillofacial Surgery. 2017;75(3):584-595. DOI: 10.1016/j.joms.2016.09.018

[163] Savage VJ, Chopra I, O'Neill AJ. *Staphylococcus aureus* biofilms promote horizontal transfer of antibiotic resistance. Antimicrobial Agents and Chemotherapy. 2013;57(4):1968-1970. DOI: 10.1128/AAC.02008-12

[164] Kulkarni R, Antala S, Wang A, Amaral FE, Rampersaud R, LaRussa SJ, et al. Cigarette smoke increases

Staphylococcus aureus biofilm formation via oxidative stress. Infection and Immunity. 2012;**80**:3804-3811. DOI: 10.1128/IAI.00689-12

[165] Wright JA, Nair SP. Interaction of staphylococci with bone. International Journal of Medical Microbiology. 2010;**300**:193-204. DOI: 10.1016/j. ijmm.2009.10.003

[166] de Mesy Bentley KL, Trombetta R, Nishitani K, Bello-Irizarry SN, Ninomiya M, Zhang L, et al. Evidence of Staphylococcus aureus deformation, proliferation, and migration in canaliculi of live cortical bone in murine models of osteomyelitis. Journal of Bone and Mineral Research. 2017;**32**(5):985-990. DOI: 10.1002/jbmr.3055

[167] de Oliveira-Neto OB, Timbó Barbosa FT, de Sousa-Rodrigues CF, de Lima JC. Quality assessment of systematic reviews regarding immediate placement of dental implants into infected sites: An overview. The Journal of Prosthetic Dentistry. 2017;**117**:601-605. DOI: 10.1016/j. prosdent.2016.09.007

[168] Friscia M, Sbordone C, Petrocelli M, Vaira LA, Attanasi F, Cassandro FM, et al. Complications after orthognathic surgery: Our experience on 423 cases. Oral and Maxillofacial Surgery. 2017;**21**:171-177. DOI: 10.1007/ s10006-017-0614-5

[169] Almadih A, Al-Zayera M, Dabela S, Alkhalafa A, Mayyada AA, Bardisi W, et al. Orthodontic treatment consideration in diabetic patients. Journal of Clinical Medicine Research. 2018;**10**(2):77-81. DOI: 10.14740/ jocmr3285w

[170] Faber J, Morum T, Jamilian A, Eslami S, Leal S. Infection predictive factors with orthodontic anchorage miniplates. Seminars in Orthododontics. 2018;**00**:00-00. DOI: 10.1053/j. sodo.2018.01.004

[171] Aly SA, Alyan D, Fayed MS, Alhammadi MS, Mostafa YA. Success rates and factors associated with failure of temporary anchorage devices: A prospective clinical trial. Journal of Investigative and Clinical Dentistry. 2018;**00**:00-00. DOI: 10.1111/ jicd.12331

[172] Tortamano A, Dominguez GC, Haddad ACSS, Nunesd FD, Nacaoe M, Morea C. Periodontopathogens around the surface of mini-implants removed from orthodontic patients. Angle Orthodontist. 2012;**82**:591-595. DOI: 10.2319/081011-506.1

[173] Kouskoura T, Katsaros C, von Gunten S. The potential use of pharmacological agents to modulate orthodontic tooth movement (OTM). Frontiers in Physiology 2017;**8** (Article 67): 1-9. DOI: 10.3389/ fphys.2017.00067

[174] Smith KF, Goldberg M, Rosenthal S, Carlson L, Chen J, Chen C, et al. Global rise in human infectious disease outbreaks. Journal of the Royal Society Interface. 2014;**11**:20140950. DOI: 10.1098/rsif.2014.0950

[175] Salomon D, Heidel RE, Kolokythas A, Miloro M, Schlieve T. Does restriction of public health care dental benefits affect the volume, severity, or cost of dental-related hospital visits? Journal of Oral Maxillofacial Surgery. 2017;**75**:467-474. DOI: 10.1016/j. joms.2016.10.019

[176] Barenghi L, Barenghi A, Di Blasio A. Infection Control in Dentistry and Drug Resistant Infectious Agents: A Burning Issue. Part 2. UK: InTech; 2018

[177] Degeling C, Johnson J, Iredell J, et al. Assessing the public acceptability of proposed policy interventions to reduce the misuse of antibiotics in Australia: A report on two community juries. Health Expectations. 2018;**21**: 90-99. DOI: 10.1111/hex.12589

[178] Rennert-May E, Conly J, Lea J, Smith S, Manns B. Economic evaluations and their use in infection prevention and control: A narrative review. Antimicrobial Resistance and Infection Control. 2018;7(31):1-6. DOI: 10.1186/s13756-018-0327-z

[179] Gao Q, Sui W. The function of nursing management for stomatology clinic infection. Journal of Nursing and Health Studies. 2017;2(1):1-4. DOI: 10.21767/2574-2825.100008

Chapter 5

Infection Control in Dentistry and Drug-Resistant Infectious Agents: A Burning Issue. Part 2

Livia Barenghi, Alberto Barenghi and Alberto Di Blasio

Abstract

We showed that antibiotic-resistant bacterial infections inside of dental settings are relevant. Here, we have focused on the limited awareness on infection prevention guidelines, and the lapses and errors during infection prevention, which sustain the evidence of possible reservoirs of antibiotic-resistant bacterial infections in humans (dental staff and patients) and on dental items or in the environment. We chose Staphylococci and Enterobacteriaceae as markers since they are considered as prioritized bacteria according to antibiotic resistance pressure, and the data are available on their virulence factors and for dental settings. For better dental patient and healthcare personnel safety, we need to improve knowledge on bioburden and biofouling, based also on molecular biological methods, and education and training initiatives to limit the hazards in surgical dental settings and to sustain accreditation survey.

Keywords: dentistry, surgery, guidelines, infection control, MRSA, biofilm

1. Introduction

Antibiotic-resistant bacterial infections inside of dental settings are relevant and nearby [1] (Part 1). The limited awareness on infection prevention guidelines, lapses, and errors during infection prevention according to Centers for Disease Control and Prevention (CDC) dental guidelines sustains the evidence of possible reservoirs of antibiotic-resistant infectious agents (ARIAs) in humans (patients and dental staff) and in the environment (clinical contact surfaces (CCSs), dental instruments, and dental unit water lines (DUWLs)) and possible hazards mainly in surgical dental settings [2–26]. Here, we have focused mainly on hand hygiene, PPE use, environment decontamination, and instrument reconditioning [19, 20, 27–29]. We focus on Staphylococci and Enterobacteriaceae as markers since they are considered as prioritized bacteria according to antibiotic resistance pressure [30], and better knowledge is available on their virulence factors (adherence to abiotic surfaces, biofilm formation, ability to growth also in anaerobic conditions) and for dental settings (i.e., contamination of hands and environments, etc.). These features are important in the exploration of standard precaution failures since bacterial adherence to inanimate objects (i.e., many objects in dental settings, dental implants, collagen-based biomaterials, etc.) is known to be linked with the presence of surface components with nonpolar/hydrophobic vs. polar/hydrophilic characteristics; in particular for methicillin-resistant *Staphylococcus aureus* (MRSA), its estimated infective dose is very low (4 CFU) [31–42]. Fast and very sensitive molecular biological techniques (quantitative real-time polymerase chain reaction (PCR), multiplex PCR, microarray, next-generation sequencing technologies, etc.) and *in vivo* biosensors technology seem to be a very promising support to improve the knowledge on bioburden and biofouling, even due to not cultivable infectious agents by classical microbiological methods, and to monitor the effectiveness of item reprocessing [43–47].

2. Approach

The electronic literature search was conducted via the PubMed and Google Scholar databases (from January 2010 up to and including April 2018) using various combinations of the following key indexing terms: (a) patient safety, (b) infection control, (c) implant, (d) endodontia, (e) sterilization, (f) reconditioning, (g) critical items, (h) semicritical items, (i) hand hygiene, (j) DUWL, (k) sharps safety, (l) personal protective equipment (PPE), (m) disinfection, (n) MRSA, (o) VRE, (p) ARIAs, (q) guidelines, and (r) cross infection. In addition, manual searches were carried out in InTech books. Then, bibliographic material from the papers has been used in order to find other or older appropriate sources. A total of 125 papers and links were found suitable for inclusion in this chapter (Part 2). Only few papers do not have a DOI or PubMed classification, but the available links by Internet and accessed date have been added.

3. Infection control implementation: a closer look on patient needs and cost/benefit advantages

Marketing and financial strategies are emerging in dentistry. Concerning both, the improvement of infection control (IC) seems to be very important when taking into account dental patient needs and the first economic evaluations. A clean and hygienic appearance of the dental office, the sterilization of the instruments, the hand hygiene, and use of PPE of dental workers are essential requirements for patients, increasingly informed about cross infection in dental settings [48–52].

The first economic evaluations have been published concerning IC implementation [53]. The implementation of IC procedures for 1 year resulted in an infection reduction of 65% at a dental clinic [54]. Chen's group reported that the simple implementation of hand hygiene resulted in a substantial advantage in the cost/benefit ratio ($ 1 invested vs. $ 23.7 saved) for the hospital [55]. The total expenses for the investigation and response, related to the first case of patient to patient transmission for HCV infection in dentistry, totaled at $ 681,859.01. For every HCV infection that can be avoided with infection prevention, the estimated savings are of $ 30,000–$ 40,000 based on treatment costs for HCV infection using antiviral drug [56].

4. Noncompliance, lapses, and errors during infection prevention according to CDC dental guidelines

Manjunath recently focused on the management of MRSA patients in the dental chair [57]. MRSA can be transmitted by a carrier state, often asymptomatic, in dental patients and dental healthcare personnel (DHCP) (by contaminated hands) or by spray and splash, contaminated items. The spread of ARIAs can be restricted following standard preventions: hand hygiene, clinical contact surface disinfection, and instrument reprocessing are particularly important [16–20, 27–29]. In addition, we must limit the contamination by using premouthwash and surgical aspirators during clinical activity.

The insufficient compliance of guidelines during infection prevention in dentistry depends on the limited awareness of the infective risk and mainly the fact that the dentist will not share the same fate of the patient in the case of an adverse event (AE), but the financial-occupational consequences can be just as serious as that of an airplane crash [5–8, 56, 58, 59]. Here, we confirm the current significant extent of violations and main noncompliance in IC observed in dental settings (**Table 1**), sadly not different from those previously reported [12–15, 60–68].

4.1 Hand and glove contamination of DHCP

In 1991, MRSA transmission was caused by ungloved hands of a dentist on two patients during dental surgery (see in [10]). Nowadays, this situation is likely to happen due to the violations or noncompliances of hand hygiene and the use of PPE (**Table 1**) as stated in the key recommendations for hand hygiene and for PPE in dental settings [3]. In addition, MRSA hand carriage rates in dental patients, nurses, and dentist were 9.8, 6.6, and 5% [21]. Staphylococci were detected in 57% samples from gloves *S. aureus* (5%), CNS (52%), *S. epidermidis* (44%), MRSA (1.5%), MRCNS (2.2%), MRS *epidermidis* (1.5%), respectively [69].

The rationale of surgical hand washing and the correct gloving is to preserve surgical glove sterility. Since the high turnover of dental patients in private practice and the need for frequent hand hygiene, alcohol-based (95% wt/wt) hand rub is recommended as a speeder alternative to surgical scrub (4–5 minutes) and to apply:

- when hands are not visibly soiled

- before donning gloves and after glove removal

- following instruction for use (IFU) (product amount, time) by the manufacturer since are efficacious on MRSA even when gloves were not used for routine clinical care [70]

- since DHCP needs short time procedures and it takes only 20–30″

- since it is safe for patients and workers [71].

Concerning gloves, the physical properties of different materials influence bacterial passage in case of glove puncture due to sharp injuries [27–29, 72]. Glove perforation was 17% in maxillofacial surgery, and occurred significantly more frequently in procedures that exceeded 90 minutes than in those taking less time or during surgical procedure with a high risk of percutaneous injury rate (long procedures: intermaxillary fixation, sinus lift), in surgeon and first assistants. In addition, endodontia and orthognathic surgery are at high risk of glove perforation [13, 73]. Needlestick and sharp injuries occur as a consequence of poor visibility, unexpected patient movements, and during the clearing up of dental instruments at the end of treatments and manual cleaning [27–29, 74]. According to the European Directive n° 32/2010 and National rules, there are a lot of key recommendations for sharps' safety and good practice guides for sharp safe dental treatment [3, 29]. Sharp injuries can be reduced to a degree by behavioral changes, training, and engineering

Study (publication date, country) [reference]	Dental setting	Hand hygiene (%)	Use of protective eyewear (%)	Use of gloves (%)	Wearing/use of mask (%)	Instrument reprocessing (%)	Autoclave quality control (%)	Handpieces reprocessing after every patients (%)	Other violations or noncompliances (%)
Hübner et al. (Germany) [60]	35 dental practices	11	15–23			6 (autoclave class N)	80	67	
Mutters et al. (Germany) [61]	58 invasive dental cares in university dental clinic	95 (N) 61–65 (D) (after glove removal)		14.3 (D♀) 28.6 (N)	16 (N)				Presence of jewelry during DP in N (80.7%)
Copello et al. (review) (Italy) [62]	76 different dental practices (dentist males (78%), professionals aged 50 years or above (59%))		40 (goggles)			2 (lack of steam autoclave class B)			DUWL: 10%: lack of any infection control; 50%: absence of analytical control of the DUWL water was carried out only in nearly half of the dental practices; 77%: absence of a microbiological assessment of the work-environment contamination. 15% of the dental practices: presence of expired pharmaceuticals; 40%: not regular stocking of waste materials
Balcheva et al. (Bulgaria) [63]	94 dental students	35.5 (prewash); 8.5 (postwash)	79.8 (goggles); 95.7 (shield)	8.5	33.0 (use); 51.1 (mask change)				

Study (publication date, country) [reference]	Dental setting	Hand hygiene (%)	Use of protective eyewear (%)	Use of gloves (%)	Wearing/ use of mask (%)	Instrument reprocessing (%)	Autoclave quality control (%)	Handpieces reprocessing after every patients (%)	Other violations or noncompliances (%)
Anders et al. (USA) [64]	214 dental students (third-fourth year)	56.8 (during the preoperative phase); 23.3 (postoperative phase after removing gloves)		53.7	35.7				12%: overall noncompliance with infection control parameters in dental students
Dagher et al. (Lebanon) [65]	1150 private dental clinics	9.9	54.3	7.6	10.9	21 (automatic washing of used instruments); 35 (steam autoclave) ; 34.7 (dry heat sterilized burs and 39.7 (dry heat sterilized endodontic files; 29.6 (wrapping barrier for instrument sterilization)		72.3	19 (wiping with disinfectant on CCSs); 44.9 (use of surface barriers); 61.6% (impression disinfection
Mandourh et al. (Saudi Arabia) [66]	107 dentists working in 34 private dental clinics in ten districts (♂: 66.4%; ♀: 33.6%)	65.4 (after glove removal (D) with the daily workload (>10 patients/day): the correct time (66.3%); correct duration (41.3%) and drying (18.8%); after removing the gloves (25%); washing with soap and water after contact with saliva (56.3%) or alcohol hand rub when hand is visibly dirty (80%)	♂:8.5; ♀: 5.6 (nonawareness of wearing protective eyewear)	54.2	11.2	Keeping sterile instruments in pouches (3.8%)		4.6	70%: unsafe work behavior of bending needles after use; 12.2%: not disposing sharps in a safety container; 2.8%: do not believe separation of blood-soaked waste is important. The incorrect practice of opening drawers with contaminated gloved hands was done by 81.3% of the dentists with daily workloads of more than 10 patients.

Study (publication date, country) [reference]	Dental setting	Hand hygiene (%)	Use of protective eyewear (%)	Use of gloves (%)	Wearing/ use of mask (%)	Instrument reprocessing (%)	Autoclave quality control (%)	Handpieces reprocessing after every patients (%)	Other violations or noncompliances (%)
Yadav et al. (India) [67]	30 dental surgeons working in a private dental hospital	50 (hand sanitizer)	93.4	5 (disposable gloves) 80 (sterile gloves)	20	66 (autoclave); ~70 (use of irritant disinfectants for instruments; 10 (bur reconditioning); 30 (endodontic files reconditioning)	10		100% (use of rubber dam); 90% (use of high speed evacuator); 100% (use of surface barriers)
da Costa et al. (Brazil) [68]	641 undergraduate dentistry students, 20 Ph.D. students, 15 oral radiology professors								Many factors in oral radiology, mainly associated with: plastic barriers, performance of infection control procedures; use of overgloves

D, dentist; N, dental nurse; DP, dental procedure; , female; , male; CCSs, clinical contact surfaces.

Table 1.
Violations or noncompliances (%) concerning selected infection control procedures.

innovations. Nevertheless, with the exception of free-standing needle guards, needle burners, blade-safe surgical blade remover, and rigid puncture-proof yellow hidden waste bin, some engineering innovations (i.e., disposable retractable scalpel blade, blunt-tip suture needles) are no longer the methods of choice or it is not proven best protection in dentistry. There is no data on the best protection and early identification of perforation of using double gloving with an indicator in dentistry [75]. Single-use gloves intended for use in nonsterile areas must meet the requirements as reported and an AQL of ≤1.5 in accordance with EN 455–1 [76]. However, Al-Swuailem found gloves with higher defect rates (as high as 20%) than what is considered acceptable (2.5%) according to the international regulations [77]. Then, we suggest extreme caution on the cheapest gloves and at lower quality of sterile gloves available in the market, as these could have unclear or fake AQL, which is crucial for glove perforation. It is not known whether *Enterococcus* hand carriage is possible in DHCP for prolonged periods [78, 79], but the glove perforation is high in endodontics also using electronic root canal length measurement devices [80].

4.2 Environmental contamination in dental setting

Nowadays, it is widely recognized that environmental surface contamination plays an important role in the transmission of healthcare-associated infections [81]. The aerosols generated by high-speed handpieces, ultrasonic scalers, air polishing, air-water syringe sprays, contaminated water from DUWL [82], patient's saliva and blood, and respiratory secretions from MRSA carriers could cause air and then CCSs and item contamination, above all when dam and surgical high-speed evacuator are not used. *Staphylococcus* and *Enterococcus* species are present in DUWL water [83]. Despite the fact that DUWL biofilm is intrinsically resistant to antibiotics, Omogbai's paper showed a wide presence of ARIAs, mainly associated to *Pseudomonas* ssp. isolates [84].

We underline the numerous violations and noncompliance concerning two aspects: (a) the use of standard surgical masks, which is risky in relation to MRSA carriers among DHCP and (b) surface disinfection [1, 21, 65] (**Table 1**). Barenghi reviewed the microbial contamination of CCSs and analyzed the guidelines, products, and procedures (barrier protective coverings, disinfectants vs. cleaners, impregnated wipes, choice of surface disinfectant and wipes) for the management of CCSs [13–15]. Here, we report some updated data focused on ARIAs.

There was no indication of a special tendency or heightened ability of MRSA to aerosolize [85]. *S. aureus*, including MRSA, can remain virulent for 10 days on dry surfaces and survive for 7 days to 9 weeks on dry inanimate surfaces and 2 days on plastic laminate surfaces, while *Enterococcus* spp., including VRE, can survive from 5 days to 4 months on dry inanimate surfaces [86–88].

Since 2006, the dental operatory had to be considered a possible reservoir of MRSA [89]. Before the revision of IC protocols, 6% of patients were infected by HA-MRSA among those hospitalized for oral and maxillofacial diseases. After treating the patients under a revised IC protocols, including single use of barrier covers, MRSA was not detected on the surfaces of the dental operatory, and no HAI occurred during hospitalization. MRSA long-term persistence in a simulation of dental operative conditions up to 4 months suggests that the risk for MRSA diffusion on CCSs is high in the dental office [90]. In fact, hydrophobic microorganisms adhere relatively easily to medical devices and CCSs constructed from hydrophobic materials (rubber, silicon, stainless steel, teflon, etc.); in addition, the bacterial attachment depends on many other factors (material topography at the micro- and nanoscale) [40–42].

The dynamics of microbial colonization among patients, staff, and inanimate surfaces are not known in dental settings [91]. A dental operative room is certainly different from a hospital room, but the turnover of patients, relatives, and DHCP could be very high, especially in orthodontic offices. The presence of ARIAs on CCSs in dental setting has been confirmed from the puzzle of different operative theaters:

- 21% of dental students and 8.4% frequently touched dental school clinic surfaces were MRSA positive [92],

- 1.3% of the environmental isolates were MRSA-positive, and there were no statistical differences in biofilm-forming ability between MRSA isolates recovered from DHCP and those recovered from environmental surfaces [21],

- 10-fold increase in viable bacteria during periods of clinical activity vs. the absence of such activity, 73 species selected and 48% of species resistant to at least an antibiotic using 16S ribosomal RNA gene sequencing [93],

- greater contamination of surfaces with MRSA colonies was observed after patients were treated in five different departments of a hospital dental clinic. High prevalence of MRSA strains has been observed on various surfaces, especially the paper dental records in the oral medicine department [94],

- MRSA prevalence rate was different in samples from dental surgery (4.3%), prosthetic dentistry (3.9%), operative dentistry (2.9%), periodontics (2.4%), prosthodontic (1%), and endodontic (0.98%). The majority of MRSA and SA isolates recovered from environmental surfaces were biofilm producers [21, 95],

- the contamination of *S. aureus* and MRSA on the gloved-dominant hand and the tray are similar, being 5 and 1.5% respectively [69],

- the more frequently contaminated items were panoramic headrest/chin rest, radiation shields, towel dispenser, keyboard, and chair arm inside patient care areas of an academic dental clinic. 4.7% of abiotic surfaces in treatment and nontreatment areas were contaminated with *S. aureus* (<5 CFUs). Most isolates were resistant to penicillin [96],

- a high contamination of SA and MRSA species have been reported from materials used in radiographic processing, mainly on the lids of the portable dark rooms [97],

- in dental settings, the phone contamination is very high and is by *S. aureus*, *E. coli*, *Enterococcus*, and *Pseudomonas* (see Ref. in [13–15, 98]),

- only a few, dental surfaces were positive for *E. faecalis* (0.9%), but on the other hand, disinfection of surfaces reduced contamination levels by only 10% [54]. After clinical activity, the microbial surface contamination by *S. aureus* and *E. faecalis* was, 20 and 10%, respectively [93], and

- widespread microbial contamination of air, surface, and dental unit water samples and violations concerning environmental cleaning have been reported in dental surgeries [17, 18].

Recommendations for assessing the effectiveness of disinfection and cleaning practices indicate that the suitable levels of total bacterial numbers in the health care setting are in the range of 2.5–5 CFU/cm^2 [99]. It has been shown that the presence of a significant total coliform contamination, as markers of the presence of feces, before surface disinfection or on some dental materials "received from manufacturer" and/or "clinically exposed" (see in Ref. [13]). MRSA contamination has been detected on 2.8% of fomites [99]. Since, we frequently touch multiuse vials containing bonds, cements, pastes, etc. with contaminated gloved hands, it is important to remember that *S. aureus* and *E. faecium* may retain viability on plastic for longer than 1 year [100]. Avoiding touching everywhere with contaminated gloved hands (i.e., inside the drawers) or contaminated hands after glove disposal and obviously before a proper hand hygiene.

4.2.1 Resistant and susceptible strain survival to surface disinfectants

In general, there was no obvious difference in survival to biocides between multiresistant and susceptible strains of *S. aureus* and *Enterococcus* spp. [101]. Biocide resistance is rare since the biocides affect multiple cellular components, and this is more of a problem for Gram-negative bacteria (i.e., *Pseudomonas*), but not for *S. aureus* [102]. Resistance problems do not emerge when efficacious surface disinfectants are used properly following instruction for use (IFU) [103]. Two tested antibiotic-resistant microorganisms (MRSA, VRE) resisted to intermediate-level disinfectants in off-label conditions [104]. Recently, seven cleaning-disinfecting wipes and sprays, based on different active ingredients, were tested for their efficacy in removal of microbial burden and proteins in hospital settings. Efficacy was tested with known Dutch outbreak strains. In general, a > 5 log10 reduction of CFU for tested wipes and sprays was obtained for all tested bacteria strains, with the exception of the hydrogen peroxide spray and VRE [105].

Today, it is important to check the products carefully, including the specific biocidal activity (i.e., spectrum and time of action) at least of the main ARIAs, you use to avoid gray-market products (i.e., without approval in accordance with European Community (EC) product directives and/or FDA requirements, defective or expired) [11]. Nevertheless, inefficient surface decontamination (improper procedures, time below the contact time, insufficient dispersal, etc.) (**Table 1**) can then allow for the survival and growth of the surviving bacterial population [54, 93, 106]. The use of disposable barrier protective coverings (DBPCs) (transparent food barriers, purpose and medical-grade barriers, adhesive barriers) is recommended in particular for more contaminated zones of instruments (curing lights, intraoral radiographic equipment, computer keyboards, multiple-use dental dispenser devices, etc.), dental chair parts (dental suction units, light arms), buttons, switches, and other materials and accessories [13–15, 107]. In the future, it will be ergonomic to increase the use of the no-touch procedures (vaporization with hydrogen peroxide, HEPA filters, etc.) and rapid systems to control environmental cleanliness above all for surgical rooms.

4.3 Dental instrument reconditioning

Poor or bad instrument reconditioning practices for critical dental items are linked to cross infection [108]. Here, we reported the failures concerning dental instrument reconditioning, which includes decontamination, cleaning, wrapping, sterilization and storage. Since many multiresistant and susceptible bacterial strains in dental settings are good biofilm producers and then survive to desiccation, and are more resistant to disinfectants than planktonic communities, afterwards, the inadequate reconditioning of reusable dental instruments can potentially increase cross infection and outbreak [22, 109]. It is very important to avoid the drying of biological fluids on instruments and long delay in reprocessing (better within 6 hr) [110]. Main violations or noncompliances concerning all phases of instrument reconditioning in dental settings (**Table 1**) are very frequent and can be classified as follows: (a) lack of resources (es steam autoclave class B, unwrapped devices, insufficient drying, autoclave quality controls, etc.); (b) cleaning difficulties, above all for manual procedures, in the case of older, more complex instruments (implant drills, trephine drills, healing abutments, high-speed handpieces, torque wrenches) and dirty instruments with biological fluids, cements, bonding, adhesive, etc.; (c) many difficulties during reprocessing of surgical drills, endodontic instruments and their accessories; (d) use of water of uncertain quality for cleaning and steam autoclave; (e) insufficient training; (f) selection of item design with difficult clean ability; (g) loss of sterility; and (h) reuse of single-use medical devices (i.e., irrigation sets) [5, 12, 13, 23–26, 38, 111–115]. MRSA was demonstrated to survive on sterile item packaging for more than 38 weeks [113]. In general, the operative problems during surgical instrument reconditioning are more frequent since instruments can be single-end sharps (elevators), heavy (forceps), and joint fit (bone chisels, scissors, forceps, suturing forceps, etc.); in addition, they often have a hole and/or a cavity or are very little and sharp (drills, trephine drills). Instruments or surgical drills made with different alloys or old or very used are particularly tricky to recondition; we have to follow IFU to avoid corrosion and discharge them when have been damaged during clinical procedure (i.e., contact between bone drill and dental periosteal elevator) and/or reconditioning (i.e., lack of compatibility, contact in ultrasonic washer) [23–26]. Surgical and dental instruments should be discharged when corrosion stains, signs of milling or grazes [116], etc., are present. Since the reported contamination on surgical drills and instrument, we have to follow IFU and use ultrasonic washer with proper cleaning products using controls [117].

The use of surgical cassettes with modern hole patterns and washer disinfector allows an optimal cleaning and thermo-disinfection of surgical instruments with little occupational risk and better efficiency and instrument integrity. Surgical cassettes have different sizes, configurations, and can be specialized to meet specific surgical needs [118]. In the case of implantology, the surgical cassette normally holds some hand instruments, drills and screwdrivers, torque ratchet, and accessories for implantology. The correct sorting of the instruments is facilitated by the color-coding markings and pictograms [119, 120]. Manufacturer's electronic information for the processing with EN ISO 17664 is available.

Another advantage of this planning is that the surgical kit is reassembled directly in the operating room, and instruments are fixed in the open position. Using WD, there are advantages of no instrument contact or rubbing, and better automatic cleaning. Routine quality control is possible by inserting appropriate controls for cleaning efficacy (wash-checks WD STF, Browne) and the moist heat process (Descheck, Browne) inside the cassette. Recently, Valeriani proposed a fast simple molecular approach (by microflora DNA analysis) for monitoring the effectiveness of item reprocessing, which seems to be a very promising support for surveillance in dental care settings [46].

5. Conclusion

The prevention of cross infection by adopting guidelines is easily applicable and has had early significant effects on infection prevention and cost saving [53, 54] compared to the delayed significant effects due to the sustainable use of antibiotics in dentistry [121]. We reported many concurrent violations and noncompliances in infection prevention, some of which could not necessarily be harmful. Nevertheless, the infective risk is usually estimated in healthy people, while vulnerable patients (children, pregnant women, elderly people, diabetic, immune-deficient, under drug treatments, etc.) are particularly susceptible to infections from opportunistic pathogens and ARIAs. Elderly people are particularly exposed since they are often on antibiotics, situations, which favor antibiotic-resistant pathogens, and frequently require implant surgery and endodontic care. The hazard for our reputation and insurance coverage is increasing with the possibility offered by molecular biology to identify dentally acquired infections [1]. Molecular biology and *in vivo* biosensors technology, to detect quorum sensing signaling molecules produced by airborne pathogenic bacteria, can prove the violations and noncompliances in dental settings and useful for accreditation surveys [43–47, 58]. Nevertheless, antimicrobial surfaces and graphene-based antimicrobial nanomaterials seem to be promising to lower cross infection [122].

Concerning IC, we need to rapidly improve the efficacy and efficiency in IC prevention by means of:

- a better knowledge-based and rule-based behavior according to guidelines

- increased training and skill-based behavior

- high proactivity & interaction & communication among DHCP

- appropriated human and economic resources

- proper time for IC prevention (hand hygiene, gloves and mask use/change, etc.)

- use of surgical facemasks designed to rapidly inactivate dentistry-associated pathogens

- DUWL water quality and the use of sterile solution for surgery [6, 7, 14]

- digital models produced by an intraoral scan to eliminate the problem of impression and high contamination of gypsum casts (i.e., MRSA: 26.7, 15.4%, 27 respectively) [123, 124]

- more automation and no-touch procedures for cleaning and disinfection

- acceptable workload-occupational stress to avoid DHCP distraction

- use of proper items with FDA and/or CE mark [11].

For future safe and patient-centered dental cares, it is crucial that we increase the professional harmonization and ergonomics of the highly complex "human-technical dental office system" [125]. For better dental patient and DHCP safety, we need to improve education and training initiatives.

Conflict of interest

L.B. had a service agreement with KerrHawe and is a consultant for Dental Trey Il Blog (http://blog.dentaltrey.it/), neither of which gave any input or financial support to the writing of this article. There is no other conflict of interest to report.

Abbreviations

AE	adverse event
ARIA	antibiotic-resistant infectious agents
AQL	accepted quality assurance level
CDC	centers for disease control and prevention
CCSs	clinical contact surfaces
DD	dental device
DHCP	dental healthcare personnel
DI	dental implant
DUWL	dental unit water line
EC	european community
HPC	heterotrophic plate count
IC	infection control
IFU	instruction for use
MRSA	methicillin-resistant *Staphylococcus aureus*
PCR	polymerase chain reaction
VRE	vancomycin-resistant *Enterococcus*

Author details

Livia Barenghi[1]*, Alberto Barenghi[1] and Alberto Di Blasio[2]

1 Integrated Orthodontic Services S.r.l., Lecco, Italy

2 Department of Medicine and Surgery, Centro di Odontoiatria, Parma University, Parma, Italy

*Address all correspondence to: livia.barenghi@libero.it

IntechOpen

References

[1] Barenghi L, Barenghi A, Di Blasio A. Infection Control in Dentistry and Drug Resistant Infectious Agents: A Burning Issue. Part 1. Rijeka: InTech; 2018

[2] Kalenderian E, Obadan-Udoh E, Maramaldi P, Etolue J, Yansane A, Stewart D, et al. Classifying adverse events in the dental office. Journal of Patient Safety. 2017;**00**:00-00. DOI: 10.1097/PTS.0000000000000407

[3] Summary of Infection Prevention Practices in Dental Settings. USA: Centers for Disease Control and Prevention; 2016. Available from: www.cdc.gov/oralhealth/infectioncontrol/pdf/safe-care2.pdf [Accessed: 06-12-2018]

[4] Reuter NG, Westgate PM, Ingram M, Miller CS. Death related to dental treatment: A systematic review. Oral Surgery Oral Medicine Oral Pathology Oral Radiology. 2016;**123**(2):194-204. DOI: 10.1016/j.oooo.2016.10.015

[5] Cleveland JL, Gray SK, Harte JA, Robison VA, Moorman AC, Gooch BF. Transmission of blood-borne pathogens in us dental health care settings. 2016 update. The Journal of the American Dental Association. 2016;**147**(9): 729-738. DOI: 10.1016/j.adaj.2016.03.02

[6] Arduino M, Miller J, Shannon M. Safe Water, Safe Dentistry, Safe Kids. Webinar: Organization for Safety Asepsis and Prevention; 2017. Available from: https://www.osap.org/page/LecturesWebinarsConf? [Accessed: 27-05-2017]

[7] Ricci ML, Fontana S, Pinci F, Fiumana E, Pedna MF, Farolfi P, et al. Pneumonia associated with a dental unit water line. The Lancet. 2012;**379**(9816): 684. DOI: 10.1016/S0140-6736(12)60074-9

[8] Ross KM, Mehr JS, Greeley RD, Montoya LA, Kulkarni PTA, Frontin S, et al. Outbreak of bacterial endocarditis associated with an oral surgery practice. The Journal of the American Dental Association. 2018;**149**(3):191-201. DOI: 10.1016/j.adaj.2017.10.002

[9] Perea-Perez B, Labajo-Gonzalez E, Acosta-Gio AE, Yamalik N. Eleven basic procedures/practices for dental patient safety. Journal of Patient Safety. 2015. DOI: 10.1097/PTS.0000000000000234

[10] Petti S, Polimeni A. Risk of methicillin-resistant *Staphylococcus aureus* transmission in the dental healthcare setting: A narrative review. Infection Control and Hospital Epidemiology. 2011;**32**(11):1109-1115. DOI: 10.1086/662184

[11] Collins FM. The significance of the US Food and drug administration for dental professionals and safe patient care. The Journal of the American Dental Association. 2017;**148**(11): 858-861. DOI: 10.1016/j.adaj.2017.08.026

[12] Oosthuysen J, Potgieter E, Fossey A. Compliance with infection prevention and control in oral health-care facilities: A global perspective. International Dental Journal. 2014;**64**(6):297-311. DOI: 10.1111/idj.12134

[13] Barenghi L, Barenghi A, Di Blasio A. Implementation of recent infection prevention procedures published by centers for disease control and prevention: Difficulties and problems in orthodontic offices. Iranian Journal of Orthodontics. 2018;**13**(1):e10201. DOI: 10.5812/ijo.10201

[14] Barenghi L. Clean, Disinfect and Cover: Top Activities for Clinical Contact Surfaces in Dentistry [Internet]; 2015. Available from: www.

kerrdental.com/resource-center/clean-disinfect-and-cover-%E2%80%93top-activities-clinical-contactsurfaces-dentistry-dr [Accessed: 06-12-2018]

[15] Barenghi L. The Daily Fight to Limit Cross-Infection in a Dental Office [Internet]. Webinar; 2017. Available from: http://blog.kavo.com/en/webinar-daily-fight-limit-cross-infection-dental-office [Accessed: 06-12-2018]

[16] Jakubovics N, Greenwood M, Meechan JG. General medicine and surgery for dental practitioners: Part 4. Infections and infection control. British Dental Journal. 2014;**217**(2):73-77. DOI: 10.1038/sj.bdj.2014.593

[17] Monarca S, Grottolo M, Renzi D, Paganelli C, Sapelli P, Zerbini I, et al. Evaluation of environmental bacterial contamination and procedures to control cross infection in a sample of Italian dental surgeries. Occupational and Environmental Medicine. 2000;**57**: 721-726. DOI: 10.1136/oem.57.11.721

[18] Schaefer MK, Michael J, Marilyn Dahl M, et al. Infection control assessment of ambulatory surgical centers. Journal of the American Medical Association. 2010;**303**(22): 2273-2279. DOI: 10.1001/jama.2010.744

[19] Rutala WA, Weber DJ; the Healthcare Infection Control Practices Advisory Committee (HICPAC). Guidelines for infection control in dental health-care settings 2003. MMVR. 2003;**52**:1-61. Available from: www.cdc.gov/mnwr/preview/mmwrhtlm/rr5217al.htm [Accessed: 06-12-2018]

[20] Rutala WA, Weber DJ, and the Healthcare Infection Control Practices Advisory Committee (HICPAC). Guideline for Disinfection and Sterilization in Healthcare Facilities; 2008. Available from: www.cdc.gov/infectioncontrol/quidelines/disinfection [Accessed: 15-02-2017]

[21] Kharialla AS, Wasfi R, Ashour HM. Carriage frequency, phenotypic and genomic characteristics of methicillin-resistant *Staphylococcus aureus* isolated from dental health care personnel, patients and environment. Scientific Reports. 2017;**7**:7390. DOI: 10.1038/s41598-017-07713-8

[22] Cheng VCCC, Wong SCY, Sridhar S, Chan JFW, Lai-Ming M, Lau SKP, et al. Management of an incident of failed sterilization of surgical instruments in a dental clinic in Hong Kong. Journal of the Formosan Medical Association. 2013;**112**:666-675. DOI: 10.1016/j.jfma.2013.07.020

[23] Hogg NJV, Morrison AD. Resterilization of instruments used in a hospital-based oral and maxillofacial surgery clinic. Journal of the Canadian Dental Association. 2005;**71**:179-182. ISSN: 1488-2159. Available from: www.cda-adc.ca/jcda/vol-71/issue-3/179.html [Accessed: 29-07-2017]

[24] Wu G, Yu X. Influence of usage history, instrument complexity, and different cleaning procedures on the cleanliness of blood-contaminated dental surgical instruments. Infection Control and Hospital Epidemiology. 2009;**30**(7):702-704. DOI: 10.1086/598241

[25] Takamoto M, Takechi M, Ohta K, Ninomiya Y, Ono S, Shigeishi H, et al. Risk of bacterial contamination of bone harvesting devices used for autogenous bone graft in implant surgery. Head and Face Medicine. 2013;**9**(3):1-5 10.1186/1746-160X-9-3

[26] Vassey M, Budge C, Poolman T, Jones P, Perrett D, Nayuni N, et al. A quantitative assessment of residual protein levels on dental instruments reprocessed by manual, ultrasonic and automated cleaning methods. British Dental Journal. 2011;**210**(9):E14. DOI: 10.1038/sj.bdj.2011.144

[27] Ehrlich T, Dietz B. Modern Dental Assisting. 5th ed. Chapter 30. USA: W.B Sounders Company; 1995. ISBN 0-7216-5053-8

[28] Miller CH, Palenik CJ. Infection Control and Management of Hazardous Materials for the Dental Team. 4th ed. Chaps. 8, 10–14, 17. Evolve. USA: Mosby Elsevier; 2010. ISBN 978-0-323-05631-1

[29] Pankhurst CL, Coulter WA. Basic Guide to Infection Prevention and Control in Dentistry. 2nd ed. Chapters 2, 4-9. UK: Wiley Blackwell; 2017. ISBN 9781119164982

[30] Centers for Disease Control and Prevention. Office of Infectious Disease. Antibiotic Resistance Threats in the United States. 2013. Available from: http://www.cdc.gov/drugresistance/threat-report-2013 [Accessed: 24-07-2018]

[31] Elias CN, Meirelles L. Improving osseointegration of dental implants. Expert Review of Medical Devices. 2010;7(2):241-256. DOI: 10.1586/ERD.09.74

[32] Duraccio D, Mussano F, Faga MG. Biomaterials for dental implants: Current and future trends. Journal of Materials Science. 2015;50:4779-4812. DOI: 10.1007/s10853-015-9056-3

[33] Pokrowiecki R, Mielczarek A, Zaręba T, Tyski S. Oral microbiome and peri-implant diseases: Where are we now? Therapeutics and Clinical Risk Management. 2017;13:1529-1542. DOI: 10.2147/TCRM.S139795

[34] Rasouli R, Barhoum A, Uludag H. A review of nanostructured surfaces and materials for dental implants: Surface coating, patterning and functionalization for improved performance. Biomaterials Science. 2018;6:1312-1338. DOI: 10.1039/c8bm00021b

[35] Miranda-Rius J, Lahor-Soler E, Brunet-Llobet L, de Dios D, Gil FX. Treatments to optimize dental implant surface topography and enhance cell bioactivity. In: Almasri MA, editor. Dental Implantology and Biomaterial Dental Implantology and Biomaterial. Rijeka: InTech; 2016. pp. 110-127. DOI: 10.5772/62682

[36] Toledo-Arana A, Valle J, Solano C, Arrizubieta MJ, Cucarella C, Lamata M, et al. The enterococcal surface protein, Esp, is involved in *Enterococcus faecalis* biofilm formation. Applied and Environmental Microbiology. 2001;**67**(10):4538-4545. DOI: 10.1128/AEM.67.10.4538–4545.2001

[37] Komiyama EY, Lepesqueur LSS, Yassuda CG, Samaranayake LP, Parahitiyawa NB, Balducci I, et al. Enterococcus species in the oral cavity: Prevalence, virulence factors and antimicrobial susceptibility. PLoS One. 2016;**11**(9):e0163001. DOI: 10.1371/journal.pone.0163001

[38] Dancer SJ. Controlling hospital-acquired infection: Focus on the role of the environment and new technologies for decontamination. Clinical Microbiology Reviews. 2014;**27**(4): 665-690. DOI: 10.1128/CMR.00020-14

[39] Petti S, Polimeni A, Dancer SJ. Effect of disposable barriers, disinfection, and cleaning on controlling methicillin-resistant *Staphylococcus aureus* environmental contamination. American Journal of Infection Control. 2013;**41**(9):836-840. DOI: 10.1016/j.ajic.2012.09.0

[40] Reifsteck F, Wee S, Wllklnson BJ. Hydrophobicity-hydrophilicity of staphylococci. Journal of Medical Microbiology. 1987;**24**:65-73. DOI: 10.1099/00222615-24-1-65

[41] Hsu LC, Fang J, Borca-Tasciuc DA, Worobo RW, Moraru CI. Effect of micro-and nanoscale topography on the

adhesion of bacterial cells to solid surfaces. Applied and Environmental Microbiology. 2013;**79**(8):2703-2712. DOI: 10.1128/AEM.03436-12

[42] Krasowska A, Sigler K. How microorganisms use hydrophobicity and what does this mean for human needs? Frontiers in Cellular and Infection Microbiology. 2014;**4**(112):1-7. DOI: 10.3389/fcimb.2014.00112

[43] Siqueira JF, Fouad AF, Rocas IN. Pyrosequencing as a tool for better understanding of human microbiomes. Journal of Oral Microbiology. 2012;**4**: 10743. DOI: 10.3402/jom.v4i0.10743

[44] Tsunemine H, Yoshioka Y, Nagao M, Tomaru Y, Saitoh T, Adachi S, et al. Multiplex polymerase chain reaction assay for early diagnosis of viral infection. In: Samadikuchaksaraei A, editor. Polymerase Chain Reaction for Biomedical Applications. Rijeka: InTech; 2016. pp. 69-82. DOI: 10.5772/65771

[45] Rozman U, Turk SŠ. PCR technique for the microbial analysis of inanimate hospital environment. In: Samadikuchaksaraei A, editor. Polymerase Chain Reaction for Biomedical Applications. Rijeka: InTech; 2016. pp. 119-134. DOI: 10.5772/65742

[46] Valeriani F, Protano C, Gianfranceschi G, Cozza P, Campanella V, Liguori G, et al. Infection control in healthcare settings: Perspectives for mfDNA analysis in monitoring sanitation procedures. BMC Infectious Diseases. 2016;**16**:394. DOI: 10.1186/s12879-016-1714-9

[47] Ibacache-Quiroga C, Romo N, Díaz-Viciedo R, Dinamarca MA. Detection and control of indoor airborne pathogenic bacteria by biosensors based on quorum sensing chemical language: Bio-tools, connectivity apps and intelligent buildings. In: Rinken T, editor. Biosensing Technologies for the Detection of Pathogens—A Prospective Way for Rapid Analysis. Rijeka: InTech; 2018. pp. 73-87. DOI: 10.5772/intechopen.72390

[48] Hiivala N. Patient safety incidents, their contributing, and mitigating factors in dentistry [thesis]. Universitatis Helsinkiensis; 2016

[49] Chang WJ, Chang YH. Patient satisfaction analysis: Identifying key drivers and enhancing service quality of dental care. Journal of Dental Sciences. 2013;**8**:239-247. DOI: 10.1016/j.jds.2012.10.006

[50] Shyagali TR, Bhayya DP. Patient's attitude and knowledge towards the usage of barrier technique by orthodontists. International Journal of Infection Control. 2012;**8**(3):1-8. DOI: 10.3396/ijic.v8i3.9667

[51] Alagil NA, Mubayrik AB. Dental patients' knowledge, awareness, and attitude regarding infection control procedures. The Australasian Medical Journal. 2017;**10**(9):789-799. DOI: 10.21767/AMJ.2017.3123

[52] Luo JYN, Liu PP, Wong MCM. Patients' satisfaction with dental care: A qualitative study to develop a satisfaction instrument. BMC Oral Health. 2018;**18**(15):1-10. DOI: 10.1186/s12903-018-0477-7

[53] Rennert-May E, Conly J, Lea J, Smith S, Manns B. Economic evaluations and their use in infection prevention and control: A narrative review. Antimicrobial Resistance and Infection Control. 2018;**7**(31):1-6. DOI: 10.1186/s13756-018-0327-z

[54] Gao Q, Sui W. The function of nursing management for stomatology clinic infection. Journal of Nursing and Health Studies. 2017;**2**(1):1-4. DOI: 10.21767/2574-2825.100008

[55] Chen YC, Sheng WH, Wang JT, Chang SC, Lin HC, Tien KL, et al.

Effectiveness and limitations of hand hygiene promotion on decreasing healthcare-associated infections. PLoS One. 2011;6(11):e27163. DOI: 10.1371/journal.pone.0027163

[56] Bradley KK. Dental Healthcare-Associated Transmission of Hepatitis C. Final Report of Public Health Investigation and Response. 2013. Available from: www.ok.gov/health2/documents/Dental%20Healthcare_Final%20Report_2_17_15.pdf [Accessed: 17-06-2018]

[57] Manjunath N, Banu F, Chopra A, Kumar P, Nishana F. Management of MRSA patients on the dental chair. International Journal of Research in Medical Science. 2017;5(8):3729-3733. DOI: 10.18203/2320-6012.ijrms20173595

[58] Clayton JL, Miller KJ. Professional and regulatory infection control guidelines: Collaboration to promote patient safety. AORN Journal. 2017;106: 201-210. DOI: 10.1016/j.aorn.2017. 07.005

[59] Antonucci A. Risk Management in Complex Organizations. In: Svalova V, editor. Risk Assessment. Rijeka: InTech; 2018. pp. 337-369. DOI: 10.5772/intechopen.70762

[60] Hübner NO, Handrup S, Meyer G, Kramer A. Impact of the Guidelines for infection prevention in dentistry (2006) by the Commission of Hospital Hygiene and Infection Prevention at the Robert Koch-Institute (KRINKO) on hygiene management in dental practices – analysis of a survey from 2009. GMS Krankenhaushygiene Interdisziplinär. 2012;7(1):1-6. DOI: 10.3205/dgkh000198

[61] Mutters NT, Hagele U, Hagenfeld D, Hellwig E, Frank U. Compliance with infection control practices in an university hospital dental clinic. GMS Hygiene and Infection Control. 2014; 9(3):1-5. DOI: 10.3205/dgkh000238

[62] Copello F, Garbarino S, Messineo A, Campagna M, Durando P, Collaborators. Occupational medicine and hygiene: Applied research in Italy. Journal of Preventive Medicine and Hygiene. 2015;56(2):E102-E110. PMCID: PMC4718353 and PMID: 26789987. Available from: www.ncbi. nlm.nih.gov/pmc/articles/PMC4718353. [Accessed: 12-06-2018]

[63] Balcheva M, Panov VE, Madjova C, Balcheva G. Occupational infectious risk in dentistry-awareness and protection. Journal of IMAB. 2015;21(4):995-999. DOI: 10.5272/jimab.2015214.995

[64] Anders PL, Townsend NE, Davis EL, McCall WDJ. Observed infection control compliance in a dental school: A natural experiment. American Journal of Infection Control. 2016;44(9):e153-e156. DOI: 10.1016/j.ajic.2016.01.036

[65] Dagher J, Sfeir C, Abdallah A, Majzoub Z. Infection control measures in private dental clinics in Lebanon. International Journal of Dentistry. 2017; 2017, 11 pages. DOI: 10.1155/2017/5057248

[66] Mandourh MS, Alhomaidhi NR, Fatani NH, Alsharif AS, Ujaimi GK, Khan GM, et al. Awareness and implementation of infection control measures in private dental clinics, Makkah, Saudi Arabia. International Journal of Infection control. 2017;13(1): 1-14. DOI: 10.3396/IJIC.v13i1.004.17

[67] Yadav BK, Rai AK, Agarwal S, Yadav B. Assessment of infection control practice in private dental hospital. International Journal of Research in Medical Sciences. 2017; 5(11):4737-4742. DOI: 10.18203/2320-6012.ijrms20174687

[68] da Costa E, Pinelli C, da Silva Tagliaferro EP, Corrente JE, Ambrosano GMB. Development and validation of a questionnaire to evaluate infection control in oral radiology. Dento Maxillo

Facial Radiology. 2017;**46**:20160338. DOI: 10.1259/dmfr.20160338

[69] Messano GA, De Bono V, Architrave R, Petti S. Environmental and gloves' contamination by staphylococci in dental healthcare settings. Acta Stomatologica Naissi. 2013;**29**:1255-1259. DOI: 10.5937/asn1367255M

[70] Jain S, Clezy K, McLaws M-L. Safe removal of gloves from contact precautions: The role of hand hygiene. American Journal of Infection Control. 2018;**xxx**:xxx-xxx. DOI: 10.1016/j.ajic.2018.01.013

[71] Pires D, Bellissimo-Rodrigues F, Pittet D. Ethanol-based handrubs: Safe for patients and health care workers. American Journal of Infection Control. 2016;**44**(8):858-859. DOI: 10.1016/j.ajic.2016.02.016

[72] Bardorf MH, Jäger B, Boeckmans E, Kramer A, Assadian O. Influence of material properties on gloves' bacterial barrier efficacy in the presence of microperforation. American Journal of Infection Control. 2016;**44**:1645-1649. DOI: 10.1016/j.ajic.2016.03.070

[73] Patel B. Infection control in the endodontic office. In: Patel B, editor. Endodontic Diagnosis, Pathology, and Treatment Planning: Mastering Clinical Practice. Switzerland: Springer International Publishing; 2015. pp. 87-101. DOI: 10.1007/978-3-319-15591-3_7

[74] Tlili MA, Belgacem A, Sridi H, Akouri M, Aouicha W, Soussi S, et al. Evaluation of surgical glove integrity and factors associated with glove defect. American Journal of Infection Control. 2018;**46**(1):30-33. DOI: 10.1016/j.ajic.2017.07.016

[75] Florman S, Burgdorf M, Finigan K, Slakey D, Hewitt R, Nichols RL. Efficacy of double gloving with an intrinsic

indicator system. Surgical Infections (Larchmt). 2005;**6**(4):385-395. DOI: 10.1089/sur.2005.6.385

[76] Kramer A, Assadian O. Indication and requirements for single–Use medical gloves. GMS Hygiene and Infection Control. 2016;**11**:1-6. DOI: 10.3205/dgkh000261

[77] Al-Swuailem AS. Prevalence of manufacturing defects in latex examination gloves used in selected dental practices in central Saudi Arabia. Saudi Medical Journal. 2014;**35**(7):729-733. PMID: 25028231

[78] Bandlish LK. Infection control: Removing the sensation. British Dental Journal. 2015;**219**:469. DOI: 10.1038/sj.bdj.2015.864

[79] Hayden MK. Insights into the epidemiology and control of infection with Vancomycin Resistant Enterococci. Clinical Infectious Diseases. 2000;**31**(4):1058-1065. DOI: 10.1086/318126

[80] Fully TLCS, de Souza Lucena EE, de Souza Dias TG, Barbalho JCM, Lucena VCF, de Araújo Morais HH. Glove perforations after dental care. Revista Gaúcha de Odontologia, Porto Alegre. 2015;**63**(2):175-180. DOI: 10.1590/1981-863720150002000062823

[81] Weber DJ, Anderson D, Rutala WA. The role of the surface environment in healthcare associated Infections. Current Opinion in Infectious Diseases. 2013;**26**(4):338-344. DOI: 10.1097/QCO.0b013e3283630f04

[82] Raghunath N, Meenakshi S, Sreeshyla HS, Priyanka N. Aerosols in dental practice-A neglected infectious vector. British Microbiology Research Journal. 2016;**14**(2):1-8. DOI: 10.9734/BMRJ/2016/24101

[83] Szymańska J, Sitkowska J. Bacterial hazards in a dental office: An update

review. African Journal of Microbiology Research. 2012;**6**(8):1642-1650. DOI: 10.5897/AJMR11.1002

[84] Omogbai OC, Ehizele AO, Sede MA. Prevalence and antimicrobial susceptibility profile of Pseudomonas spp isolated from water specimen in a Nigerian dental practice. Nigerian Journal of Restorative Dentistry. 2017; 2(1):16-20. Available from: https:// nisord.org/wp-content/uploads/2018/ 03/omogbai.pdf [Accessed: 23-06-2018]

[85] Hall DL. Methicillin-resistant *Staphylococcus aureus* and infection control for restorative dental treatment in nursing homes. Special Care in Dentistry. 2003;**23**(3):100-107. PMID: 14650558

[86] Mertz D, Frei R, Jaussi B, Tietz A, Stebler C, Fluckiger U, et al. Throat swabs are necessary to reliably detect carriers of *Staphylococcus aureus*. Clinical Infectious Diseses. 2007;**45**(4):475-477. DOI: 10.1086/520016

[87] Siani H, Maillard JY. Best practice in healthcare environment decontamination. European Journal of Clinical Microbiology and Infectious Diseases. 2015;**34**:1-11. DOI: 10.1007/ S10096-014-2205-9

[88] Esteves DC, Pereira VC, Souza JM, Keller R, Simões RD, Winkelstroter Eller LK, et al. Influence of biological fluids in bacterial viability on different hospital surfaces and fomites. American Journal of Infection Control. 2016;**44**: 311-314. DOI: 10.1016/j.ajic.2015.09.033

[89] Kurita H, Kurashina K, Honda T. Nosocomial transmission of MRSA via the surfaces of the dental operatory. British Dental Journal. 2006;**201**(5): 297-300. DOI: 10.1038/sj.bdj.4813974

[90] Petti S, De Giusti M, Moroni C, Polimeni A. Long-term survival curve of methicillin-resistant *Staphylococcus aureus* on clinical contact surfaces in

natural-like conditions. American Journal of Infection Control. 2012;**40**:1010-1012. DOI: 10.1016/j.ajic.2011.11.020

[91] Lax S, Sangwan N, Smith D, Larsen P, Handley KM, Richardson M, et al. Bacterial colonization and succession in a newly opened hospital. Science Translational Medicine. 2017;**9**(24):1-11. DOI: 10.1126/scitranslmed.aah6500

[92] Roberts MC, Soge OO, Horst JA, Ly KA, Milgrom P. Methicillin-resistant *Staphylococcus aureus* from dental school clinic surfaces and students. American Journal of Infection Control. 2011;**39**: 628-632. DOI: 10.1016/j.ajic.2010.11.007

[93] Decraene V, Ready D, Pratten J, Wilson M. Air-borne microbial contamination of surfaces in a UK dental clinic. The Journal of General and Applied Microbiology. 2008;**54**(4): 195-203. PMID: 18802318

[94] Faden A. Methicillin-resistant *Staphylococcus aureus* (MRSA) screening of hospital dental clinic surfaces *Staphylococcus aureus* (MRSA) screening. Saudi Journal of Biological Sciences. 2018;**xxx**:xxx-xxx. DOI: 10.1016/j.sjbs.2018.03.006

[95] Korkut E, Uncu AT, Sener Y. Biofilm formation by *Staphylococcus aureus* isolates from a dental clinic in Konya, Turkey. Journal of Infection and Public Health. 2017;**10**:809-813. DOI: 10.1016/j.jiph.2017.01.004

[96] Trochesset DA, Walker SG. Isolation of *Staphylococcus aureus* from environmental surfaces in an academic dental clinic. The Journal of the American Dental Association. 2012; **143**(2):164-169. PMID: 22298558

[97] Dos Santos RM, Dos Santos FLM, Ramacciato JC, Junqueira JLC. Evaluation of antimicrobial contamination and resistance to *Staphylococcus aureus* collected from radiographic materials used in dentistry.

Revista Gaúcha de Odontologia. 2012;
60(4):467-477. ISSN 1981-8637

[98] Fard RH, Fard RH, Moradi M,
Hashemipour MA. Evaluation of the cell
phone microbial contamination in
dental and engineering schools: Effect of
antibacterial spray. Journal of
Epidemiology and Global Health. 2017;
xxx:xxx-xxx. DOI: 10.1016/j.
jegh.2017.10.004

[99] Gerba CP, Lopez GU, Ikner LA.
Distribution of bacteria in dental offices
and the impact of hydrogen peroxide
disinfecting wipes. The Journal of
Dental Hygiene. 2016;90(6):354-361.
PMID: 29118156

[100] Heller LC, Edelblute CM. Long-
term metabolic persistence of gram-
positive bacteria on health care-relevant
plastic. American Journal of Infection
Control. 2018;46:50-53. DOI: 10.1016/j.
ajic.2017.07.027

[101] Neely AN, Maley MP. Survival of
enterococci and staphylococci on
hospital fabric and plastic. Journal of
Clinical Microbiology. 2000;38:724-726.
PMID: 10655374

[102] Poole K. Mechanisms of bacterial
biocide and antibiotic resistance. Journal
of Applied Microbiology. 2002;92:55S-
64S. PMID: 12000613

[103] Gebel J, Exner M, French G,
Chartier Y, Christiansen B, Gemein S,
et al. The role of surface disinfection in
infection prevention. GMS Hygiene and
Infection Control. 2013;8(1):1-12. DOI:
10.3205/dgkh000210

[104] Meade E, Garve M. Efficacy testing
of novel chemical disinfectants on
clinically relevant microbial pathogens.
American Journal of Infection Control.
2018;46:44-49. DOI: 10.1016/j.
ajic.2017.07.001

[105] Kenters N, Huijskens EGW, de Wit
SCJ, van Rosmalen J, Voss A.
Effectiveness of cleaning-disinfection
wipes and sprays against multidrug-
resistant outbreak strains. American
Journal of Infection Control. 2017;45:
e69-e73. DOI: 10.1016/j.ajic.2017.04.290

[106] Vidana R, Sillerström E, Ahlquist
M, Lund B. Potential for nosocomial
transmission of Enterococcus faecalis
from surfaces in dental operatories.
International Endodontic Journal. 2015;
48(6):518-527. DOI: 10.1111/iej.12342

[107] Multiple-Use Dental Dispenser
Devices [Internet]. 2017. Available
from: www.fda.gov/MedicalDevices/
ProductsandMedicalProcedures/
DentalProducts/ucm404472.htm
[Accessed: 17-06-2018]

[108] Perçin D. Sterilization practices
and hospital infections: Is there a
relationship? International Journal of
Antisepsis Disinfection Sterilization.
2016;1(1):19-22. DOI: 10.14744/
ijads.2016.76476

[109] Motamedi MHK, Navi F, Valai N,
Ghaffari K, Ardalan A. Can oral debris
on dental instruments harbor organisms
from disinfection? Journal of Oral
Hygiene and Health. 2016;4:1. DOI:
10.4172/2332-0702.1000195

[110] Li XL, Ji GY. Evaluation of the
direct relationship between bacterial
load on contaminated stainless steel
surgical instruments and the holding
time prior to disinfection and also to
analyse the efficacy of different
disinfecting solutions. Biomedical
Research. 2017;28(10):4680-4687. ISSN
0970-938X

[111] Dietze B, Rath A, Wendt C,
Martiny H. Survival of MRSA on sterile
goods packaging. The Journal of
Hospital Infection. 2001;49(4):255-261.
DOI: 10.1053/jhin.2001.1094

[112] Campbell C, Barton A, Boyle R,
Tully V. Improving the inspection and
manual cleaning of dental instruments

in a dental hospital. BMJ Quality Improvement Reports. 2016;**5**(1): u205075.w2305. DOI: 10.1136/ bmjquality.u205075.w2305

[113] Cuny E. The use of a process challenge device in dental office gravity displacement tabletop sterilizers. American Journal of Infection Control. 2015;**43**(10):1131-1133. DOI: 10.1016/j. ajic.2015.05.044

[114] Sonntag D, Martin E, Raab WHM. Representative survey on the reprocessing of endodontic instruments in Germany. British Dental Journal. 2016;**220**:465-469. DOI: 10.1038/sj. bdj.2016.333

[115] Wadhwani C, Schonnenbaum TR, Audia F, Chung KH. In-vitro study of the contamination remaining on used healing abutments after cleaning and sterilizing in dental practice. Clinical Implant Dentistry and Related Research. 2016;**18**(6):1069-1074. DOI: 10.1111/ cid.12385

[116] Barenghi L. Strumenti Danneggiati? Cause, Conseguenze e Consigli Operativi [Internet]. Available from: https://blog.dentaltrey. it/strumenti-danneggiati-cause-conseguenze-e-consigli-operativi/ [Accessed: 17-06-2018]

[117] Di Blasio A, Barenghi L. Pitfalls of cleaning controls in ultrasonic washers. American Journal of Infection Control. 2015;**43**:1372-1381. Available from: http://dx.doi.org/10.1016/j. ajic.2015.08.020

[118] Surgical cassette [Internet]. Available from: https://www.hu-friedy. com/instrument-management/ cassettes/signature-series-cassettes/signature-series-oral-surgery-cassette [Accessed: 17-06-2018]

[119] Surgical-cassette [Internet]. Available from: http://www. thommenmedical.com/en/for-clinicians/instruments-biomaterials/surgical-cassette-.html [Accessed: 17-06-2018]

[120] NobelActive/NobelParallel CC PureSet Tray [Internet]. Available from: https://store.nobelbiocare.com/it/it/ kits/pur0200# [Accessed: 17-06-2018]

[121] Degeling C, Johnson J, Iredell J, et al. Assessing the public acceptability of proposed policy interventions to reduce the misuse of antibiotics in Australia: A report on two community juries. Health Expectations. 2018;**21**: 90-99. DOI: 10.1111/hex.12589

[122] Zeng X, Wang G, Liua Y, Zhang X. Graphene-based antimicrobial nanomaterials: Rational design and applications for water disinfection and microbial control. Environmental Science: Nano. 2017;**12**:2248-2266. DOI: 10.1039/c7en00583k

[123] Egusa H, Watamoto T, Abe K, Kobayashi M, Kaneda Y, Ashida S, et al. An analysis of the persistent presence of opportunistic pathogens on patient-derived dental impressions and gypsum casts. The International Journal of Prosthodontics. 2008;**21**(1):62-68. PMID: 18350950

[124] Dawood A, Marti Marti B, Sauret-Jackson V, Darwood A. 3D printing in dentistry. British Dental Journal. 2015; **219**(11):521-529. DOI: 10.1038/sj. bdj.2015.914

[125] Mokdad M, Abdel-Moniem T. New paradigms in ergonomics: The positive ergonomics. In: Korhan O, editor. Occupational Health. Rejika: InTech; 2017. pp. 1-22. DOI: 10.5772/66393